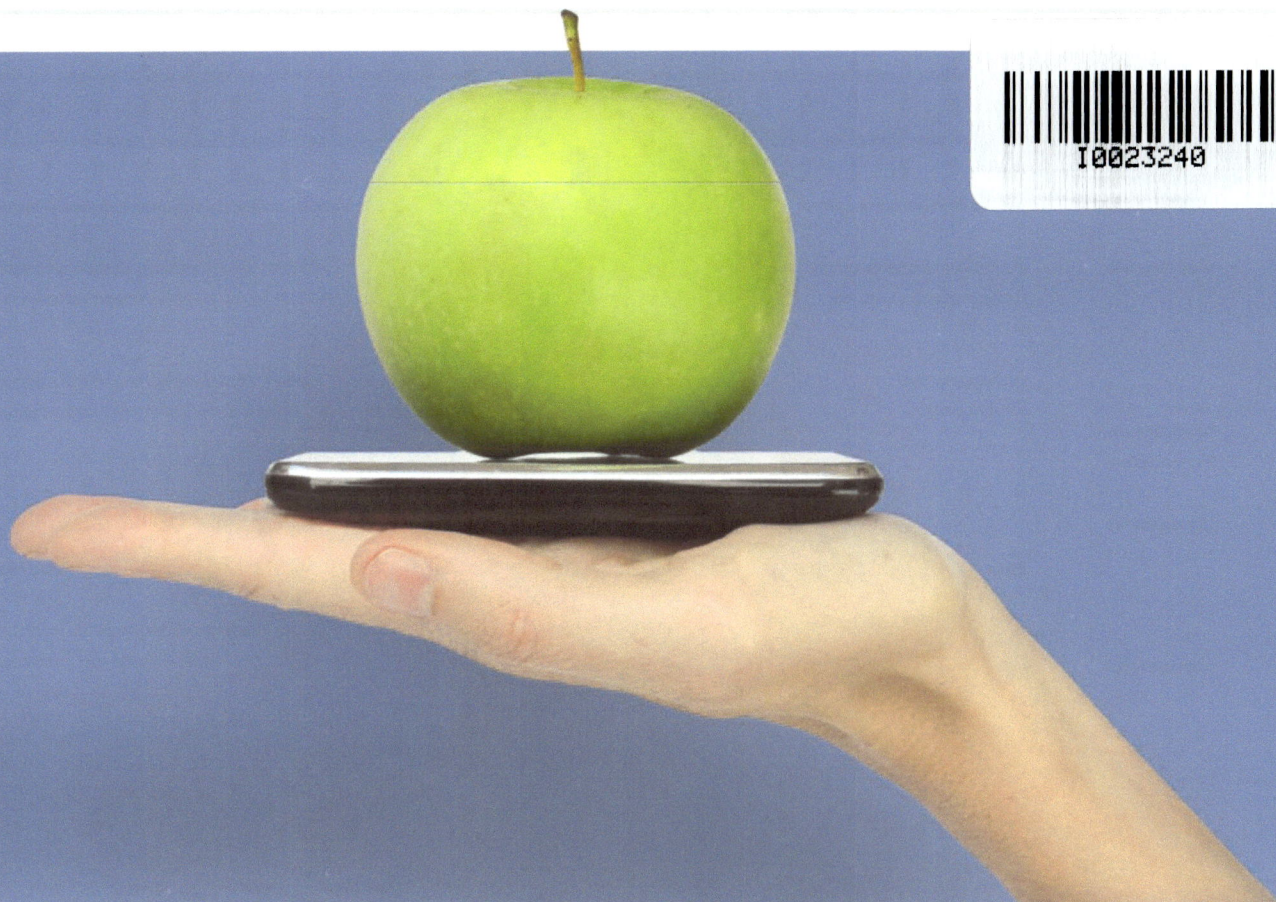

THE FUTURE OF HEALTHCARE:
IT'S HEALTH, THEN CARE

CSC Leading Edge Forum

Frances J. Turisco

CSC
Falls Church, Virginia, USA

CSC
3170 Fairview Park Drive
Falls Church, Virginia, 22042
United States

Published by Computer Sciences Corporation (www.csc.com),
printed and distributed by Lulu (www.lulu.com).

ISBN 978-0-578-07598-3

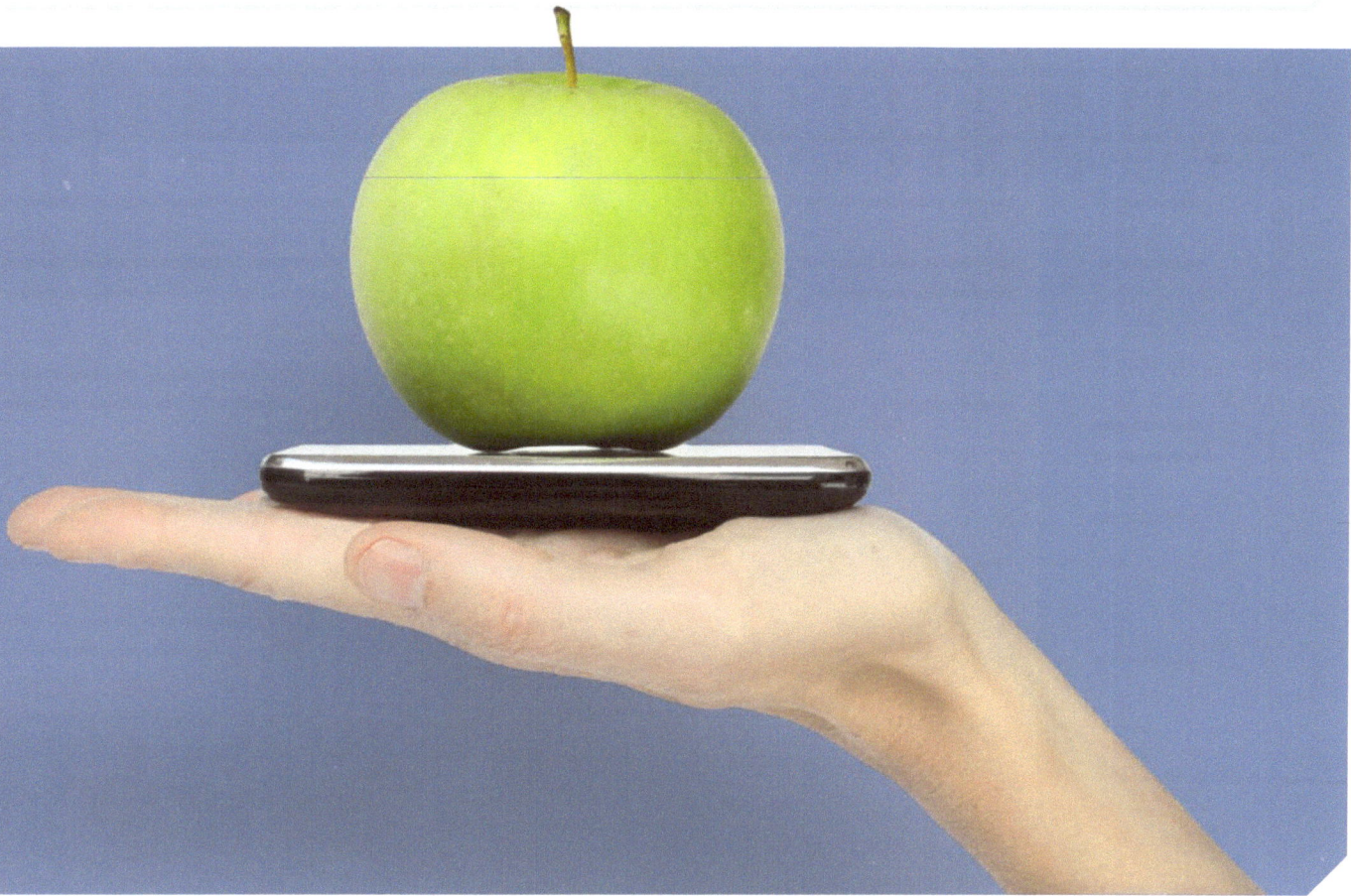

THE FUTURE OF HEALTHCARE:
IT'S HEALTH, THEN CARE

As part of CSC's Office of Innovation, the Leading Edge Forum (LEF) is a global community whose programs help participants realize business benefits from the use of advanced IT more rapidly.

LEF members work to spot key emerging business and technology trends before others, and identify specific practices for exploiting these trends for business advantage. Members enjoy access to a global network of thought leaders and leading practitioners, and to a powerful body of research and field practices.

LEF programs give CTOs and senior technologists the opportunity to explore the most pressing technology issues, examine state-of-the-art practices, and leverage CSC's technology experts, alliance programs and events. LEF programs and reports are intended to provoke conversations in the marketplace about the potential for innovation when applying technology to advance organizational performance. Visit www.csc.com/lef.

The LEF Executive Programme is a premium, fee-based program that helps CIOs and senior business executives develop into next-generation leaders by using technology for competitive advantage in wholly new ways. Members direct the research agenda, interact with a network of world-class experts, and access topical conferences, study tours, information exchanges and advisory services. Visit www.lef.csc.com.

ABOUT CSC: GLOBAL LEADER IN HEALTH

CSC delivers business and clinical consulting, process, technology and outsourcing solutions to the healthcare industry worldwide and is the largest healthcare systems integrator. CSC has approximately 94,000 employees worldwide, with more than 6,000 professionals dedicated to healthcare. Serving public, private, and not-for-profit healthcare providers, health plans, pharmaceutical companies, medical device manufacturers and allied health industries, CSC is recognized as a leader in transforming the healthcare industry through the effective use of information to improve healthcare outcomes, decision making and operating efficiency.

CSC has more than 20 years of experience in the healthcare industry, with clients in the Americas, Europe, Asia and Australia. CSC currently manages the largest eHealth initiative worldwide for the National Health Service (NHS) in the United Kingdom, reaching 15 million people and 1,300 clinics and hospitals. CSC also serves 14 of the world's top 20 pharmaceutical manufacturers, and is building and operating national and regional health information exchanges in the United States and in the United Kingdom, Denmark, The Netherlands and several other European nations. Visit www.csc.com/health_services.

LEF LEADERSHIP

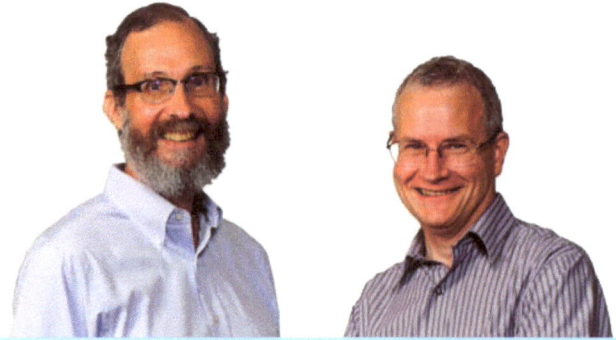

WILLIAM KOFF (LEFT)
Vice President and Chief Technology Officer, Office of Innovation

A leader in CSC's technology community, Bill Koff provides vision and direction to CSC and its clients on critical information technology trends, technology innovation and strategic investments in leading edge technology. Bill plays a key role in guiding CSC research, innovation, technology thought leadership and alliance partner activities, and in certifying CSC's Centers of Excellence and Innovation Centers. wkoff@csc.com

PAUL GUSTAFSON (RIGHT)
Director, Leading Edge Forum

Paul Gustafson is an accomplished technologist and proven leader in emerging technologies, applied research and strategy. Paul brings vision and leadership to a portfolio of LEF programs and directs the technology research agenda. Astute at recognizing how technology trends interrelate and impact business, Paul applies his insights to client strategy, CSC research, leadership development and innovation strategy. pgustafs@csc.com

In this ongoing series of reports about technology directions, the LEF looks at the role of innovation in the marketplace both now and in the years to come. By studying technology's current realities and anticipating its future shape, these reports provide organizations with the necessary balance between tactical decision making and strategic planning.

The Future of Healthcare has been produced in collaboration with CSC's global healthcare think tank, Emerging Practices. Its primary role is to understand regulatory, demographic, scientific and technology trends and then predict their impact on the health delivery, health plan and life sciences industries.

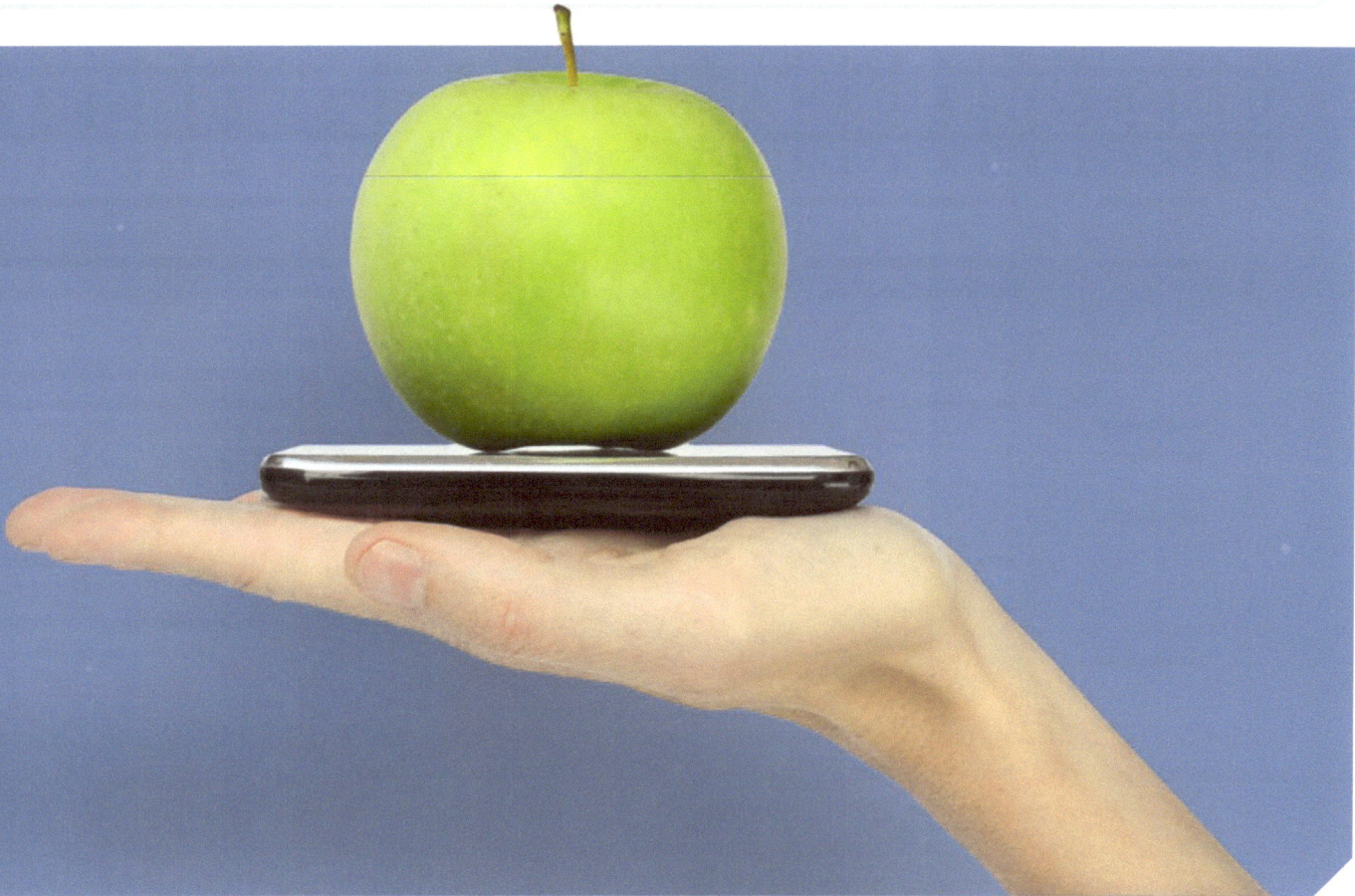

THE FUTURE OF HEALTHCARE: IT'S HEALTH, THEN CARE

You can access this report via the LEF RSS feed www.csc.com/lefpodcast or the LEF Web site www.csc.com/lefreports

WELLNESS FIRST

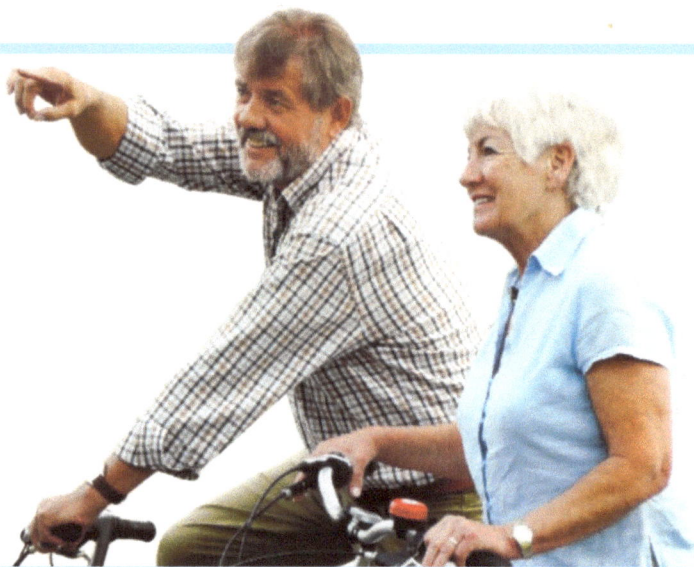

Imagine healthcare designed, first and foremost, around being well and staying healthy. Of course, people *will* get sick at times and require medical attention, but a focus on wellness shifts the balance from reactive to proactive, with better outcomes. It also expands the healthcare service continuum beyond diagnosis and treatment to include wellness monitoring, prevention and earlier disease detection.

This is a significant shift from the physician-centric model of care that has been in place since the 1860s.[1] When people did not feel well they saw their doctor, and if necessary they got further care in a hospital setting. This model worked when little was known about prevention and what causes health problems, there were few tests for detection of problems, and physicians had limited options that could help treat health issues. However, advances in medicine on all fronts make this model outdated.

"Our antiquated healthcare policies, technologies, and business models are locking us into a 19th century medical mentality that won't work for us in a 21st century economy so challenged by Global Aging," asserts Eric Dishman in U.S. Senate testimony.[2]

Today's environment demands a new approach that is both efficient and effective. Although "wellness first" is not new, its renewed focus *is* because it relieves many of the burdens of today's strained healthcare system: insufficient healthcare resources, increased demand due to an aging population, new regulatory requirements, expectations for high quality and safety, lower insurance payments, and an increasing population that is overweight and living with chronic conditions.

> The wellness-first perspective will impact patients, providers, business models and the global healthcare ecosystem as all shift to focus first on health, then on care.

Welcome to the future. The wellness-first perspective will impact patients, providers, business models and the global healthcare ecosystem as all shift to focus first on health, then on care. Advances in the practice and science of medicine will provide the next level of wellness and healthcare management, expanding life expectancy and improving the quality of life into the coming decades.

In the future of healthcare, the *practice* of medicine (how treatment is delivered) follows a care team model with new roles and new members, where wellness comes first, then early detection, and then more effective, medically-advanced treatments.

The model relies on technology to put medical knowledge and advice – once the sole purview of physicians – into the hands of patients to proactively monitor health and wellness. Technologies also change the interactions between clinicians and patients via online patient and physician communities and virtual providers, and empower changes in their roles. The success of this model is critically dependent on behavioral, educational, process and payment changes.

Role changes for individuals are one of the most difficult aspects of the transition. However, mobile technology and sensors can ease the transition by playing the role of the techno-medical assistant and constant data provider, respectively.

The *science* of medicine continues to make great strides for disease detection and treatment. Powerful prosthetics, diagnostic and treatment implants, and personalized medicine are just a few examples of how new disruptive technologies are pushing the boundaries of what medicine can and will do.

This report examines the future of healthcare through the lens of disruptive and enabling technologies, taking a holistic view and putting the patient at the center. Although business changes are not addressed per se, they are recognized as a critical component of healthcare change.

HOW DID HEALTHCARE GET TO THIS POINT?

Ironically, many healthcare problems stem from past successes. People are living longer (see Figure 1) thanks to medical treatment advances, development of vaccines that prevent diseases such as typhoid and rubella, improved healthcare for mothers and babies, safer and more nutritious foods, clean water, and improvements in the general standard of living. Long ago, the average life expectancy in Classical Greece and Rome was 28 years and in Medieval Britain it was 30.[4] In Colonial America the life expectancy was under 25 years in the Virginia Colony, and in New England approximately 40 percent of children did not reach adulthood. Today 51 countries, including the United States, European Union countries, Australia, Canada, Japan and parts of China, boast life expectancy of 78 years or more.[5] Worldwide, life expectancy is 68.[6]

However, the Industrial Age and now the Information Age have changed people's lifestyles to be more sedentary and more profitable, allowing them to have more while physically doing less. In addition, today's lifestyle of busy two-income families has changed eating habits and diets, with a plethora of companies promoting fast food and processed foods, not healthy options. In the United States alone, 66 percent of adults do not engage in physical activities regularly[7] and 61 percent of adults are overweight or obese.[8] Globally, the World Health Organization (WHO) reported as of 2005:

- Approximately 1.6 billion adults (age 15+) were overweight
- At least 400 million adults were obese
- At least 20 million children under the age of 5 were overweight

WHO also projected that by 2015, approximately 2.3 billion adults will be overweight and more than 700 million will be obese.[9]

With the combination of living longer and not staying physically fit, people are experiencing more chronic diseases and getting serious illnesses like cancer later in life. This leads to higher use of healthcare resources.

U.S. LIFE EXPECTANCY AT AGE 0
(by Sex and Calendar Year, based on Cohort Tables)

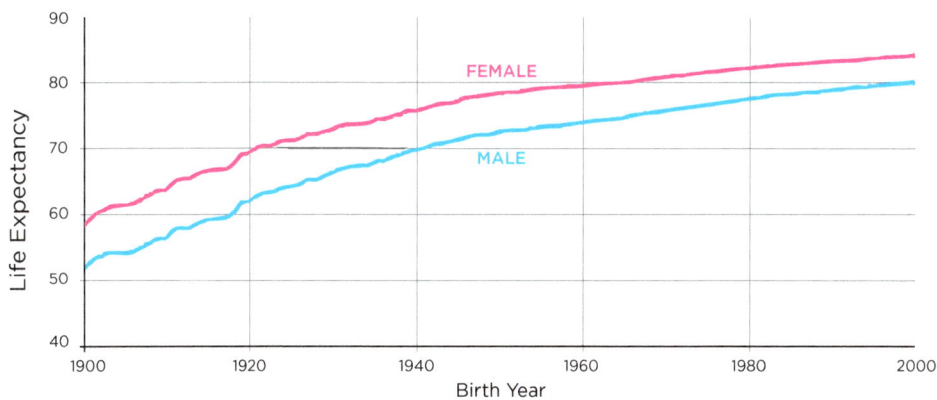

Figure 1 U.S. life expectancy grew significantly from 1900 to 1940 and continues to rise, though it has been leveling off.

Source: U.S. Social Security Administration[3]

All of these factors have significant health and financial ramifications, resulting in a health system that is being crushed under the weight of its problems:

- *Growing aging population.* From 2000 to 2050, the number of people on the planet ages 60 and over will triple from 600 million to 2 billion.[10]

- *Shortage of care providers.* By 2025, it is estimated that the United States alone will be short 260,000 registered nurses and at least 124,000 physicians.[11]

- *Increasing prevalence of chronic conditions among children and adults.* For example, diabetes for all age groups worldwide is expected to increase from 2.8 percent in 2000 to 4.4 percent by 2030.[12] By 2030 chronic diseases, not infectious diseases, will be the leading cause of death globally.[13]

- *Fragmented care management.* Only 56 percent of adult chronic condition patients in the United States receive recommended care.[14]

- *Rising healthcare costs.* For almost 50 years, spending has grown by two percentage points in excess of GDP growth across all Organisation for Economic Co-operation and Development (OECD) countries.[15] U.S. healthcare costs are expected to rise to $4.5 trillion by 2019, up from $2.5 trillion in 2009 and $2.3 trillion in 2008.[16] Research by the Australian Institute for Health and Welfare estimates the total health and residential aged care expenditure to increase 189 percent over 30 years (2003-2033), from $85 billion to $246 billion.[17]

The simple fact is that healthcare needs significant disruptive changes to address its major problems.

DISRUPTING HEALTHCARE

Fortunately, changes are already in progress. There are a myriad of burgeoning efforts in laboratories, in pilot studies, in clinical trials and in practice. The changes these efforts represent, and the implications of the key technologies involved, are presented in the context of five major trends that are disrupting healthcare. The trends focus first on patient-centric initiatives and then on new developments, care providers, and finally the emerging global ecosystem:

- *E-Power to the Patient* — The patient is in charge of his or her care management on a daily basis, marked by "shared care" between patient and provider. The patient is empowered through the availability of health information, new technologies and a support system to encourage and monitor progress.

- *Earlier Detection* — Accelerating early diagnosis is crucial to starting treatment for, if not preventing, a problem. Supporting technologies range from simple, inexpensive paper lab tests to genetic testing for variants aligned to known health problems.

- *High-Tech Healing* — Solutions can improve care and the long-term quality of life. Next-generation implants and ingestibles use a number of technologies to monitor disease progress, dispense medications, and assist and replace malfunctioning organs and limbs.

- *Resources: More, but Different* — Expertise is optimized and spread. Care provider roles change and resources are more available through remote technologies and online communities, for both care/consultation and teaching/training.

- *Global Healthcare Ecosystem Emerges* — A rich ecosystem, armed with a treasure trove of data and knowledge, supports connected care and research collaborations to advance disease identification and treatment.

Collectively, the efforts and technologies described in these trends are moving the healthcare system from a care-first to a health- and wellness-first perspective, involving more resources and leveraging a plethora of data and knowledge to advance health and research. ∎

E-POWER TO THE PATIENT

Patients take on a larger, more active role in managing their wellness and health.

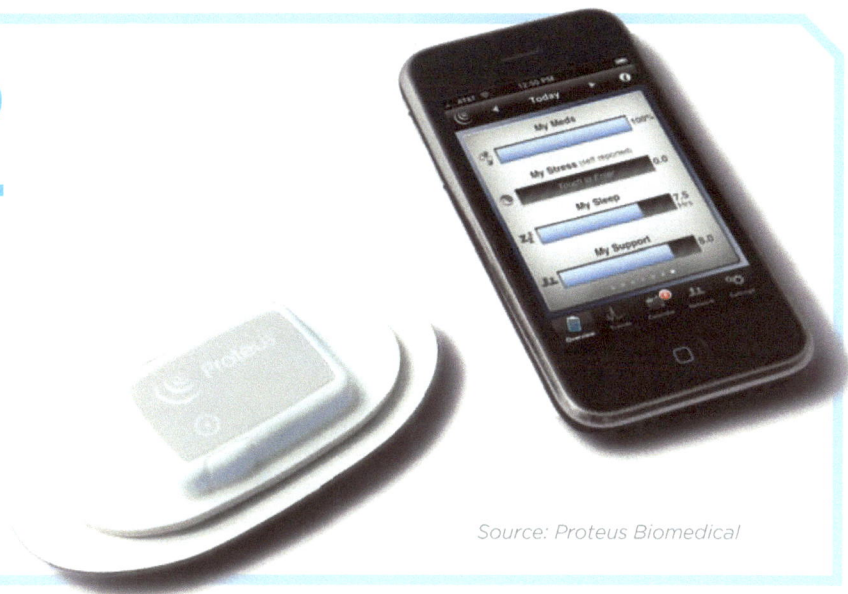

Source: Proteus Biomedical

In the past, healthcare has been a top-down proposition, with the physician at the top as sole authority instructing the patient, who played a more or less passive role. This interaction is changing as patients take on a larger, more active role in managing their wellness and health.

In this new world, the patient is in charge of his or her care management on a daily basis, with "shared care" between patient and provider; the patient and primary care provider determine a health and wellness plan together and pull in resources as needed. This is not about diminishing

the role of the physician but enlarging the role of the patient, who is empowered through changes in behavior and the use of health information bolstered by new technologies. This chapter examines this sweeping new empowerment in broad terms and how it applies to people

> This is not about diminishing the role of the physician but enlarging the role of the patient, who is empowered through changes in behavior and the use of health information bolstered by new technologies.

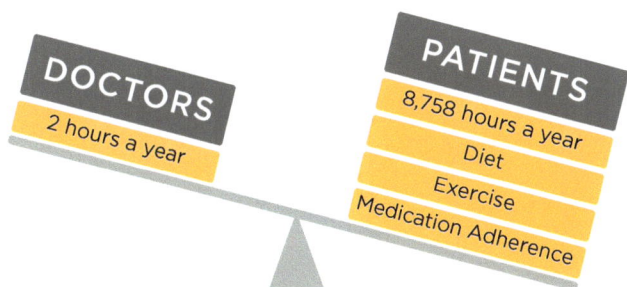

in all phases of health, including post-hospital discharge patients and the elderly.

ACTIVE PATIENT INVOLVEMENT WORKS

When looking at time spent on care management, it is clear that patients should take active roles in their care. They already make most of the treatment plan decisions regarding diet, exercise and medications. (See Figure 2.) However, although the focus on wellness and patient-centric care has been around for some time, it has had very limited success. Yet research and pilot studies show that active patient involvement does work.

DOCTORS
2 hours a year

PATIENTS
8,758 hours a year
Diet
Exercise
Medication Adherence

Figure 2 Nearly all healthcare decisions are already made by patients.

Source: CSC (data from Clayton Christensen et al, The Innovator's Prescription: A Disruptive Solution for Health Care, 2009)

For example, a recent blood pressure study conducted by Kaiser Permanente in collaboration with the American Heart Association followed 348 patients, ages 18 to 85, with uncontrolled blood pressure.[18] The participants were assigned to either the usual care group or the home monitoring group. The home monitoring group used a blood pressure device that uploaded data to that patient's personal health record. The Kaiser clinical pharmacists monitored the reading and consulted with the patients to adjust their medication levels based on proven protocols. The usual care group had their blood pressure checked during office visits. At six months, the at-home monitoring group was 50 percent more likely to have their blood pressure under control.

Health plans and self-insured employers have also taken steps to help individuals get and stay healthy. They offer risk assessments to help consumers understand their health status and provide incentives to take active steps. For example, some cover health club membership, others eliminate annual check-up co-pays, and others offer discounts on premiums if patients participate in health programs. While some success has been attained, they have been in pilot stages or have been operational for a short time.[19]

Meanwhile, for years individuals have been aware of, and willing to spend money for, fitness and health programs. Weight Watchers and similar diet programs are a $60 billion business. Health and wellness businesses are making upwards of $100 billion. What all have found is that success is short-lived unless the individual's behavior is changed to build health and fitness into his or her daily routine and to know what to do when potential health problems arise.

GETTING PATIENTS TO BE ACTIVE: SOCIAL NETWORKING

One key element of behavior change, and one where technology can play a major role, is the ability to connect with others with similar health issues for support and advice. The LEF's 2008 *Digital Disruptions* report explored how the Internet, and more specifically social networking, provides the knowledge and the connectivity with others to attain higher levels of success.[20] This includes supporting long-term behavioral changes. Social networking in the form of fitness and health Web sites – even within the boundaries of a company – and interactions such as "The Biggest Loser" weight loss contests (on TV and the Web) can bring people together to encourage and keep the motivation going.

Weight Watchers, Jenny Craig and many other programs offer Web site options that provide content, customized diets, online coaching and chat rooms. In healthcare, content Web sites such as WebMD and disease-specific Web sites with content, advice and chat rooms number in the thousands. These sites have been incredibly successful in connecting patients with medical issues to others who can share treatments, symptoms and resources, helping patients learn about available products, services and research. These sites empower the patient to proactively learn more about the disease or chronic condition. More importantly, the connections made with other patients provide encouragement to continually manage the disease, bolstered by advice on both traditional and non-traditional therapies.

One well-known site is PatientsLikeMe.com, which provides information on symptoms and treatments and then links them to known diseases. (See Figure 3.) It is the launching pad that takes the person to a disease-specific site such as one for multiple sclerosis (MS),

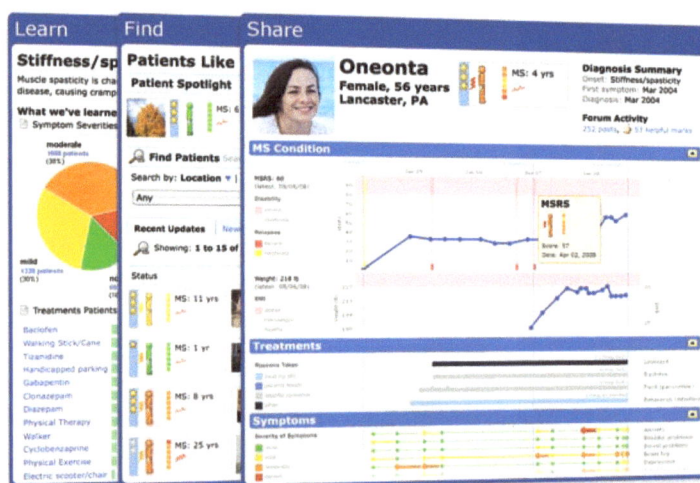

Figure 3 Health-oriented social networking sites like PatientsLikeMe.com provide information, real-world experiences and encouragement.

Source: PatientsLikeMe

where the person can connect with other PatientsLikeMe members with MS. Other healthcare social networking sites offer more than connections and content. Dlife.com for diabetics provides recipes, healthy eating recommendations, expert Q&A, diabetic supplies, news and research in addition to disease information and community support.

"The smartphone, with its apps, is the disruptive technology for patient self-care management."
—Erica Drazen, CSC

In addition to these third-party social networks, providers are tapping social networks to educate their patients. Dr. Jeff Livingston, a physician practicing in Irving, Texas, uses Facebook and Twitter to direct patients to articles and blog posts of interest. The more patients are educated, the more prepared they are for their appointment and the more engaged they are in their own care. As Dr. Livingston told *Computerworld*, "If you allow your patients to become engaged in their own health care, they ironically make really good decisions. I think that's a new concept for a lot of people."[21]

INFORMATION WHEREVER YOU ARE: THE SMARTPHONE

Many people are mobile and need their health and fitness information, encouragements and reminders wherever they are. Internet-enabled smartphones that can run applications are filling this gap. While other Internet-accessible devices are useful for home and office, the obvious advantage of the smartphone is that it's with you *all the time*. For example, one diabetic emphatically states that he often forgets his glucometer (and therefore has several) but he is never without his smartphone.

Thus, for today's patient-consumer, the device of choice is the smartphone, notably the iPhone, Android and BlackBerry. The iPhone alone has more than 5,800 health and wellness applications that can be downloaded to provide content, tracking, alerts and reminders to log vital signs.[22] Some offer options to connect to coaches, dieticians and other advisors.

"The smartphone, with its apps, is the disruptive technology for patient self-care management," says Erica Drazen, Healthcare Emerging Practices managing director at CSC. It provides new information and tools to manage health and patient behavior that never existed before. The everyday, always-with-you smartphone offers continuous access and support, with varying levels of

technology sophistication and patient-specific customization depending on the application and device configuration. Categories of functions and features include:

- *General Content* — Information for a general audience that targets the wellness objective. This includes tips for quitting smoking, dieting and administering first aid.

- *Customized Content* — Information specific to the service and individual. This includes personalized meal plans, medication schedules and exercise regimens.

- *Push Messages* — Reminders, motivational messages and alerts when there is a clinical problem.

- *Data Capture* — Activity data such as fitness activities, vital signs and other patient information. Data are stored and can be trended over time.

- *Interactive Services* — Advice and recommendations such as food selections, location of the closest emergency room, and direct communication with care professionals. Data are sent from the device to a central repository and other clinical systems.

A few examples from the abundance of established and emerging patient self-management solutions illustrate how these features apply to fitness monitoring, medical content and medical advice, and monitoring and treatment. These solutions, available on smartphones and the Web, help to put patients in control of their health.

Boost Health and Fitness. Taking results from a metabolic assessment (done at one of their centers), iNewLeaf makes an iPhone a fitness tracker with the addition of its Digifit Connect device and Digifit app suite. (See Figure 4.) During customized, guided

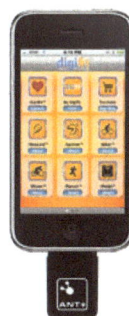

Figure 4 Exercisers can turn their iPhone into a fitness tracker using the Digifit app suite and Digifit Connect device, which attaches to the phone and collects data wirelessly from nearby health and fitness sensors.

Source: New Leaf

workout sessions, the iPhone records heart rate, time in target zones, total calories expended, cadence, speed, distance, and power, and issues zone alerts (to change intensity).[23] Pedal Brain has a similar attachment and app for cyclists and includes a GPS location function viewable online.[24]

Medical Content and First Aid. WebMD, now mobile, provides medical information on demand – symptoms, medications, treatment information and basic first aid instructions. HealthWise, a nonprofit provider of health materials and knowledge bases, specifically targets consumers by avoiding medical jargon and is used by a number of health apps such as WebMD.[25]

Similarly, iTriage provides medical information, advice and treatment locations wherever the consumer may be located. It was developed by two emergency room physicians who saw a need for patients to have actionable healthcare information at their fingertips. iTriage has information on more than 300 symptoms, 1,000 diseases and 250 medical procedures. It includes a directory of hospitals, urgent care facilities, retail clinics, pharmacies and physicians. iTriage can also link directly to TelaDoc, a national network of board certified physicians (www.teladoc.com), as well as nurse hotlines, so the consumer can get advice from a provider on the spot. (See Figure 5.)

Health Monitoring and Treatment. What if a person's heart rate could be checked regularly by simply wearing a Band-Aid? The U.S. Food and Drug Administration (FDA) recently approved Proteus Biomedical's wireless adhesive sensor technology, called Raisin, which can track and record a patient's heart rate, physical activity, body position and other biometrics. Raisin, which is worn like a Band-Aid, then transmits the data via Bluetooth to a PC or mobile device. (See Figure 6.) This eliminates physician office visits to check heart rates, and since they are monitored continuously, adverse events can be spotted right away.

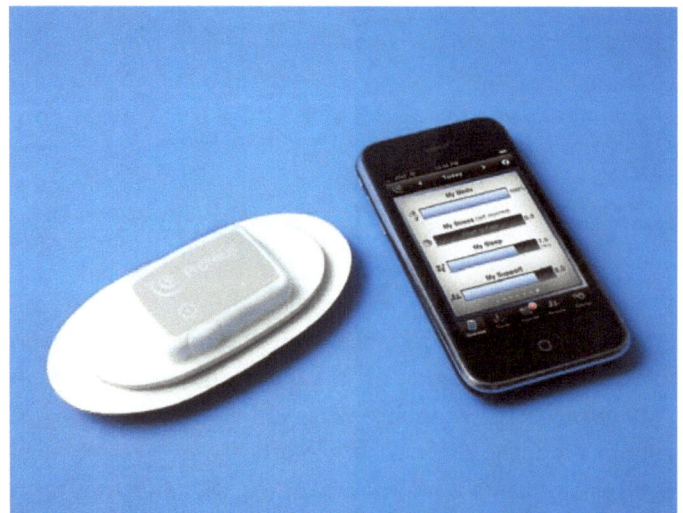

Figure 6 People can monitor their heart rate continuously with this Band-Aid-like sensor, called Raisin, which transmits data wirelessly to a mobile device or PC.

Source: Proteus Biomedical

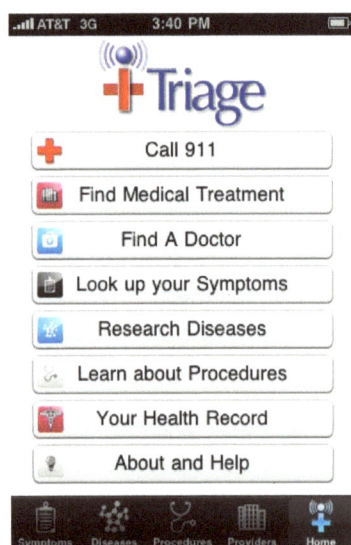

Figure 5 iTriage puts medical information at people's fingertips.

Source: Healthagen

Raisin is just one part of the intelligent medicine system that aims to link "sensor-based formulations of pharmaceutical products to individualized physiologic response and outcomes-based treatment systems."[26] The other key part of the system is a smart pill for tracking medication adherence. (See High-Tech Healing.)

LET'S GET EVERYONE INVOLVED

The solutions cited thus far are singular in that they focus on one aspect of fitness or care such as diet, fitness, disease identification or health monitoring. They are extremely useful and help address the continuous observation component of a wellness-first approach.

However, what is missing is a holistic closed-loop team solution for wellness and health management. This involves a cadre of health, wellness and family members connected using technologies that share data, provide knowledge and alert team members when an event (that is relevant and important to them) has occurred.

Figure 7 depicts how patient empowerment and technology work hand in hand in a team solution (described in more depth in Resources: More, but Different).

The technology core is a self-care solution that has a suite of wellness and health applications to advise, monitor alerts and connect team members. Although there are no total solutions currently in place, there are a number of well-funded studies and emerging commercial products and services on the horizon. (For an example of how such a solution would work, see the scenario about Ann on page 12.)

E-POWER TO THE PATIENT POST-HOSPITALIZATION

Following treatment for a hospitalized health condition, post-acute patients need intensive monitoring of vital signs or other condition-specific measures to speed recovery and avoid re-admission. In the past, health delivery organizations have piloted the use of nurse transition coaches, who call patients and make house calls to help them understand medication changes, arrange follow-up appointments, and ensure that patients are keeping up with therapy or dietary requirements. While the results of these studies show positive outcomes,[27] this labor-intensive approach is typically not done due to lack of available resources and cost.

The future healthcare system eliminates barriers by using a technology-enabled, patient-interactive approach. The technology reminds the patient to enter daily vital sign and health information, sends the data, analyzes the findings, and alerts transition coaches and care providers only when patients need their help. For post-acute care the smartphone is not typically the patient device of choice; it is an Internet-connected home PC with medical devices attached to help the patient collect vital signs. (See the scenario about Mildred on page 13.)

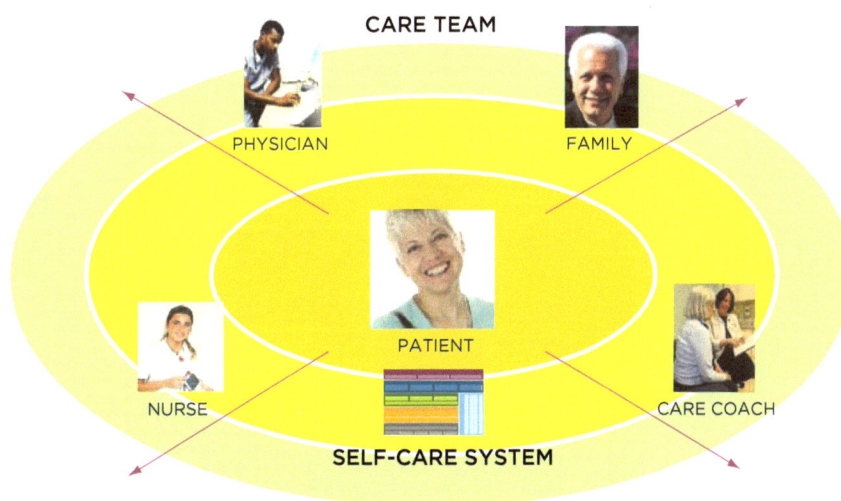

CARE TEAM

PHYSICIAN

FAMILY

PATIENT

NURSE

CARE COACH

SELF-CARE SYSTEM

Figure 7 The patient is at the center of a team-based "wellness first" solution. Information is shared among patients, physicians, nurses, care coaches and family members.

Source: CSC (Adapted from Chris Zook, Beyond the Core, *2004)*

MEET ANN,
WHO MANAGES HER DIABETES THROUGHOUT THE DAY

Ann Smith is a 46-year-old advertising executive with type 2 diabetes. She starts her day by checking key vital signs before breakfast. She weighs herself and then measures her blood glucose level. Her devices are wirelessly connected to her home PC, which automatically sends the data to the patient self-care system.

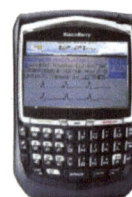

The system receives Ann's data and compares the values to her benchmarks and the care protocol set up by Ann and her physician. Ann's values are within normal ranges, so the system sends an acknowledgment to Ann's smartphone and reminds her to take her morning medications. Using her smartphone, she records that she took her medications. Throughout the day the system reminds Ann to check her vital signs and gives her feedback.

TECHNOLOGY SUMMARY
- Medical devices collect data and send to home PC.
- Home PC sends via Internet to self-care system.
- System applies logic to determine patient's health status.

- System sends message back to Ann.
- Data sent to care coach and doctor's office (weekly).
- Smartphone sends monitoring reminders and collects data from patient direct entry.

PATIENT BENEFITS
- Keeps blood sugar in control
- Avoids complications of diabetes
- Stays active and can maintain current lifestyle and work life while managing a chronic disease

Ann

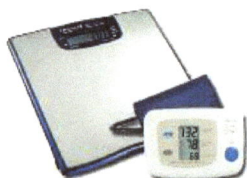

Wireless scale and blood pressure cuff send data

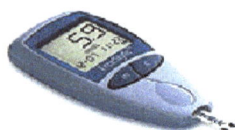

Wireless glucose monitor sends data

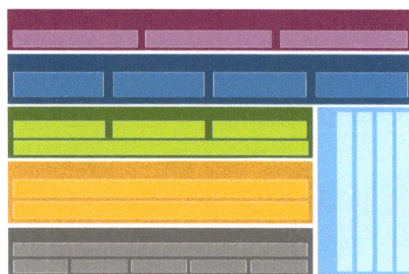

Self-Care System

Ann receives acknowledgment on her smartphone

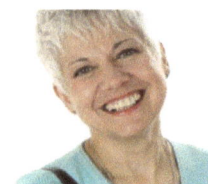

MEET MILDRED,
A RECENTLY DISCHARGED PATIENT WHO MONITORS HER HEALTH AT HOME

Mildred is an active 72-year-old woman with congestive heart failure and hypertension. She has just been discharged from the hospital and has been taught how to use her new home monitoring devices, including a digital blood pressure cuff. Each day she takes her vital signs and answers a few questions about how she feels. She can also view educational videos at her convenience.

The information is sent to a third-party monitoring application. Based on her data and survey responses, Mildred may be told to contact her physician or to go to the emergency department. Data are sent to her cardiologist's electronic health record, her primary care physician's electronic health record, and her own personal health record.

TECHNOLOGY SUMMARY

- Devices record the date and time patients take medications, complete education sessions and take vitals.

- The home monitoring system receives incoming data, applies the escalation logic, and communicates with recipients as needed.

- Data are sent to a call center or physician's office if medications are missed or if patient data indicate the patient is having problems.

- Selected data are sent to the physician's electronic health record and the patient's personal health record.

PATIENT BENEFITS

- Receives daily feedback on health status and progress

- Can review personalized patient education and clinical content

- Keeps her physicians aware of her health status

- Stays at home to recuperate without readmission to the hospital

Mildred

▶

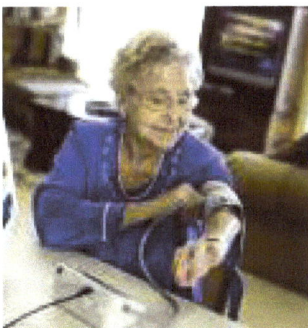

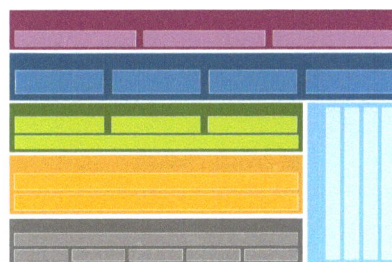

Self-Care System

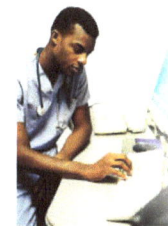

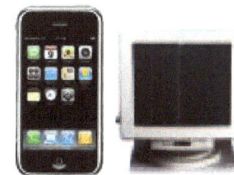

▶

Automated phone message sent for missed medications or abnormal vital signs

E-POWER TO THE AGING PATIENT

As people continue to age, technology in the home plays a larger role. Monitoring is intensified, and sophisticated logic "knows" the person's routine and can send alerts when changes occur. Multi-level monitor systems use visual, sound and motion sensors that collect patient data without the awareness of the person being monitored.

One example of passive monitoring is the smart toilet, which monitors urine sugar levels during a regular bathroom visit. The toilet is one "health smart" device in the Intelligence Toilet II bathroom jointly developed by Toto and Daiwa House Industry Co. This high-tech bathroom

As people continue to age, technology in the home plays a larger role.

includes a special scale and blood pressure cuff so people can also monitor weight, body-mass index and blood pressure on a regular basis. Data from all devices is transmitted via Wi-Fi to a home computer for analysis. This type of tracking makes it easy for people to keep abreast of changing body conditions thanks to regular, convenient monitoring. (See Figure 8.)

Throughout the home, all health sensor devices are connected to the home's local area network, which is connected to a home computer. A key application on the home computer is the patient's electronic personal health record, which stores all information to provide a total health picture. Patient information is also transmitted through the Internet to the patient's professional caregivers (e.g., nurses, nurse aides, service coordinators, elder care managers) and potentially to the patient's informal caregivers, such as family members and friends who provide assistance.

Living Laboratories. Two organizations that have taken a leading role in healthcare and the digital medical home, promoting "aging in place" technologies, are the Technology Research for Independent Living Centre (TRIL), in Dublin, Ireland, and the Oregon Center for Aging and Technology (ORCATECH). Both groups use interdisciplinary teams of ethnographers, designers and engineers to investigate new technologies in people's homes for living independently. These "living labs" enable researchers to observe how people interact with the technology at home and how to best design the technology for optimal adoption. (See Figure 9.)

The goal is to prevent the loss of independence among the aging and infirm by detecting early warning signs and mitigating, if not preventing, the problem.

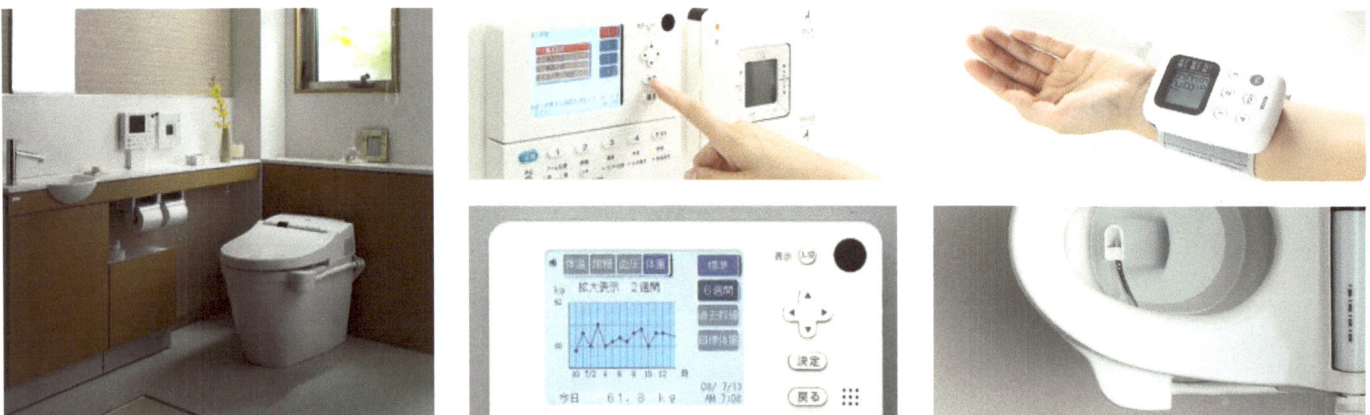

Figure 8 The Intelligence Toilet II bathroom enables people to monitor their health at home. The bathroom's smart toilet, scale and blood pressure cuff record urine sugar levels, weight, body mass index and blood pressure, transmitting the data via Wi-Fi to a home computer for analysis.

Source: Toto and Daiwa House Industry Co.

"The living lab concept in practice at TRIL and ORCATECH is central to our research philosophy," explains Steve Agritelley, director of product research and innovation in Intel's digital health group. (Intel co-founded TRIL and is a major funder of ORCATECH.) "We study people in their home settings, discover unmet needs and then build and test solutions to meet those needs – all in people's homes. This people-centered process provides a much greater chance of 'getting it right' – of discovering solutions that could add value to people's lives and are fun and easy to use. Our vision of aging-in-place solutions is to provide choice, support personalized care, and ease the burden on our over-institutionalized healthcare system," Agritelley says.

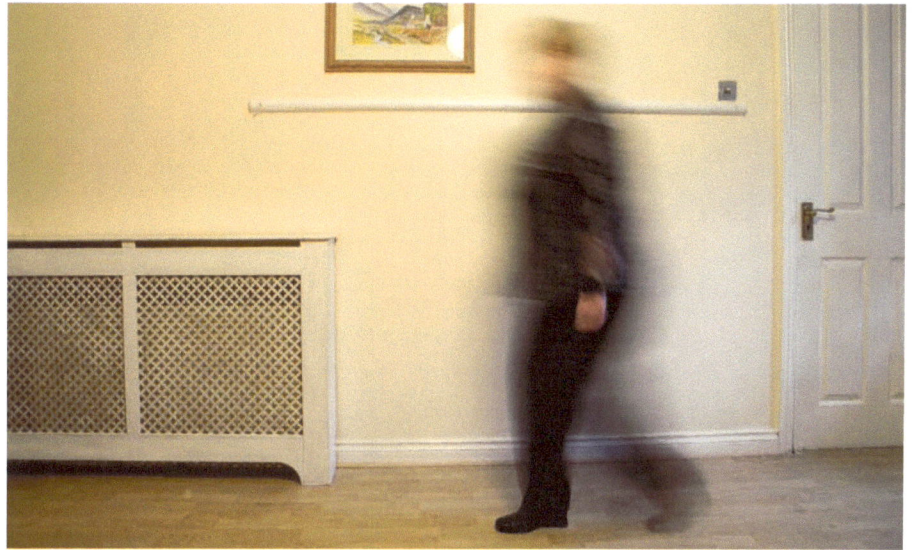

Figure 9 Hallway sensors in the home (in the white bar below the picture frame) monitor walk speed to help detect and prevent imminent falls.
Source: TRIL Centre

E-POWER MEANS MORE E-DATA

The shift to patient-centric care and continuous monitoring ushers in a wealth of new data that are collected and shareable. As people take a more active role in their wellness and care, they collect and send out more and more personal health data. Although outside of the scope of this report, numerous processes, policies and technologies need to be in place to support the patient's decisions related to data privacy, security and access.

While these and other issues are addressed, e-power to the patient presses on. As patients gather and share more personal health data, they get better at monitoring their health, maintaining wellness, and detecting medical problems earlier on. ∎

EARLIER DETECTION

Earlier detection maximizes options for successful treatment, leading to a speedier return to good health.

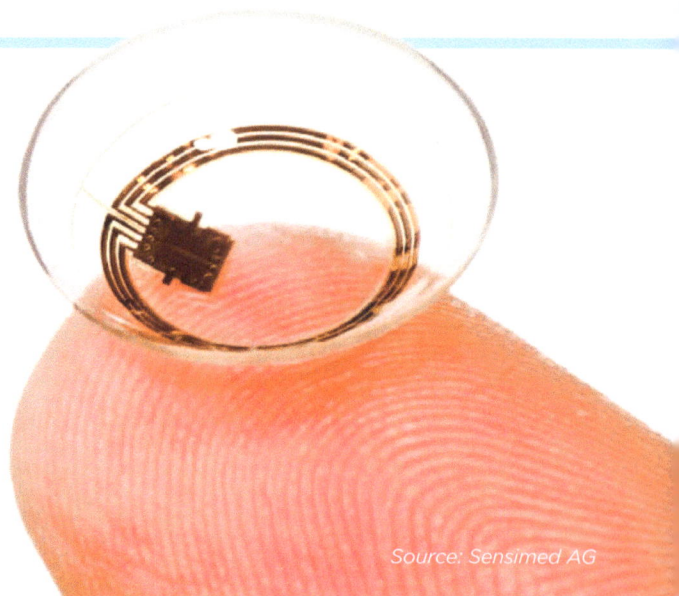

Source: Sensimed AG

According to Clayton Christensen in his book *The Innovator's Prescription: A Disruptive Solution for Health Care,* the core goals that a new healthcare system should seek are simplicity, affordability and access for all.[28] Diagnostic solutions using sensors, radio frequency identification (RFID), miniaturized electronics, nanotechnology and computer-analyzed DNA sequencing not only exemplify Christensen's core goals, which result in a better outcome for the patient,

With new detection technologies, serious conditions such as glaucoma, diabetes and digestive system problems can be mitigated, if not entirely avoided.

but will ultimately result in substantial reduction in healthcare costs. With new detection technologies, serious conditions such as glaucoma, diabetes and digestive system problems can be mitigated, if not entirely avoided.

PATIENT STARTS THE PROCESS

Detection starts with the patient – a person knows when something is not right health-wise. Now armed with a library of medical content written especially for non-clinical professionals, many people start on the Internet with sites such as iTriage, WebMD and ADAM. According to the U.S. Centers for Disease Control and Prevention,

"From January through June 2009, 51 percent of adults aged 18-64 had used the Internet to look up health information during the past 12 months."[29] As discussed in E-Power to the Patient, the Internet has gone mobile and so has the content – including GPS navigation to the nearest physician or clinic if the person feels that the illness needs immediate attention.

The patient, however, is not a physician. Therefore, the next step when there is a health problem is to seek professional help. Fortunately, physicians and their staff are equipped with new technologies that help them detect problems quicker, with less pain and wait time for the patient, and with the same or better results. These technologies are often simpler to use, less expensive, and more broadly available than previous methods.

EASIER, CHEAPER, FASTER

The camera pill is an example of a diagnostic test that is an easier and cheaper alternative to undergoing surgery to detect problems within the gastrointestinal system. Designed at the University of Washington, the camera pill can be used to detect early signs of esophageal cancer, the fastest growing cancer in the United States.[30] Instead of the traditional endoscope, a flexible camera about the width of a human fingernail that is inserted down the esophagus, patients swallow a pill that contains the camera. Using an endoscope requires sedation; the pill does not.

Using nanotechnology, Sotiris Pratsinis, a professor at the Swiss Federal Institute of Technology, Zurich, has developed a breath sensor able to detect very high acetone levels, an indicator of diabetes.[31] (Diabetics typically have twice the level of acetone as non-diabetics.) The sensor is also able to diagnose ketoacidosis, a dangerous insulin deficiency indicated by especially high levels of acetone in the breath. The device, shown in Figure 10, contains

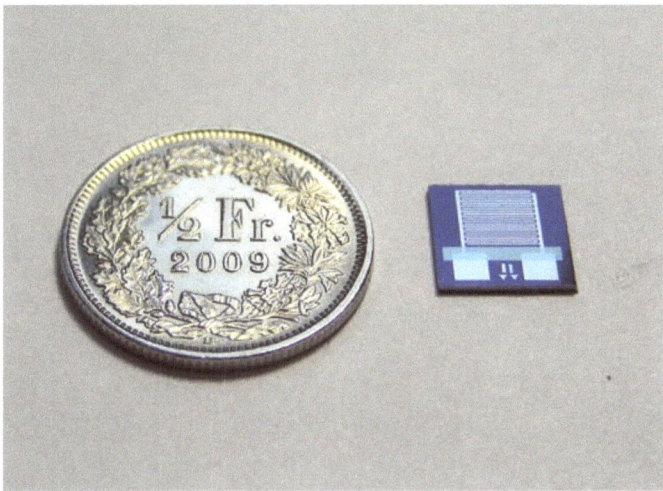

Figure 10 This tiny sensor uses nanotechnology to detect diabetes by measuring acetone levels in a person's breath. Instead of taking a blood test, just breathe.

Source: ETH Zurich

ceramic nano-particles deposited between a set of gold electrodes that act like an electrical resistor. Acetone-filled air causes the resistance to lessen and more electricity to pass through the electrodes. While the breath of a healthy person causes little change in the resistance, the breath of a diabetic patient causes it to suddenly drop. In the future this technology may be used at home for daily insulin measurements, eliminating finger pricking.

A typical diagnostic method for detecting diabetes requires patients to stop eating and drinking for eight hours before undergoing a blood test. For a definitive diagnosis, this test should be performed at least twice. A different method requires a patient to ingest a glucose drink and then have blood drawn at repeated intervals. Both are much more costly and time consuming for the patient than a breath test.

A breath test has also been devised for detecting cancer. Analyzing volatile organic compounds (VOCs) to detect cancer is a new frontier because it is non-invasive and potentially inexpensive. These VOCs can be detected through exhaled breath, as cancer-related changes in the blood chemistry lead to measurable changes in the breath. A tailor-made array of cross-reactive sensors based on gold nanoparticles can discriminate between breath VOCs of healthy patients and those suffering from lung, prostate, breast and colorectal cancers. The test, in development, is fast, easy to carry out and does not necessarily require a trained operator – all leading to more widespread screening and earlier detection.[32]

In the area of sleep disorders, sleep apnea is a chronic condition that disrupts sleep three or more nights a week as breathing pauses or becomes shallow, resulting in significant daytime sleepiness. It is currently diagnosed in specialized sleep clinics, where the patient sleeps under observation for one to two nights at a cost up to $4,000. Given the cost and inconvenience, most patients do not go to a clinic until the problem is severe.

Watermark Medical has developed and received approval from the FDA for a new at-home sleep apnea monitoring device and Web service. The sensor-equipped headband measures 10 vital signs including blood-oxygen saturation, air flow, pulse rate and snoring. The patient wears the device for one or two nights and returns the device to the physician's office. The data

The cancer-detecting breath test, in development, is fast, easy to carry out and does not necessarily require a trained operator – all leading to more widespread screening and earlier detection.

are downloaded and sent to sleep professionals, who deliver a report, within two days, that includes diagnosis and treatment. The test costs from $250-$450.[33]

Not only is the test cheaper, it is much more convenient and easier to do for the patient. If a technology is easier for the patient – less invasive, lightweight, convenient – the patient is more likely to have the test done, and earlier rather than later. Identifying, monitoring and managing from an early stage will prevent more catastrophic conditions later on.

MORE ACCESSIBLE

Coupled with simpler and cheaper, technologies must be more accessible to more people to facilitate early detection. In poor rural areas, diagnostic tests made of paper can be used to screen for multiple diseases and conditions. (See Figure 11.) A drop of blood or urine from the patient on a specially-treated square of paper sets off a reaction that shows up as varying colors on the paper, indicating different conditions. Inexpensive to make and use, the postage-stamp-size tests are small, rugged, versatile and easy to dispose of.[34] They are ideally suited for poor rural areas where people may not have consistent access to adequate healthcare. Harvard researcher George Whitesides, who developed the paper tests, envisions them being used to detect, for example, liver problems in people in Africa. He also wants to develop tests for diseases such as tuberculosis, malaria and HIV.[35]

Another example of an upcoming early testing technology that is less expensive, easier and faster is an off-the-shelf digital camera device that is powerful enough to allow physicians to distinguish between cancerous and healthy tissue. (See Figure 12.) Rice University biomedical engineers and researchers from the University of Texas M.D. Anderson

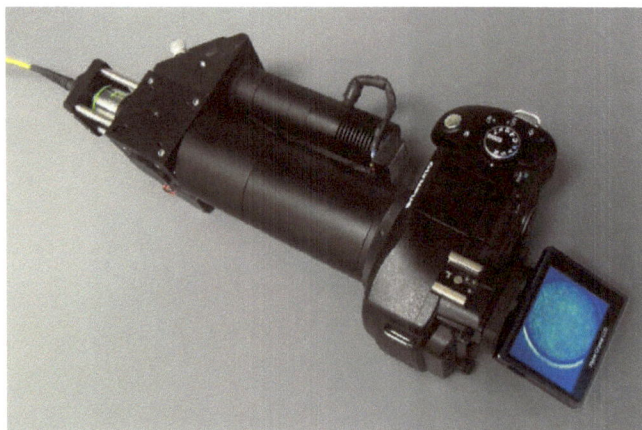

Figure 12 Using an off-the-shelf camera and a fiber-optic cable, researchers have created a faster, cheaper way to detect cancerous tissue by looking at pictures of the cells on the camera.

Source: Dongsuk Shin

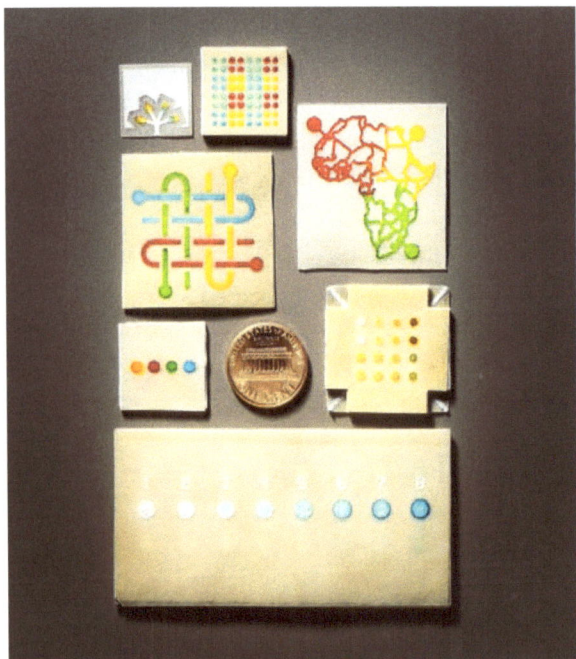

Figure 11 Inexpensive diagnostic tests made of paper can be widely distributed, making early detection accessible to vast numbers of people, especially those in developing countries.

Photo Source: Bruce Peterson

Cancer Center have captured images of cells with a small fiber-optic cable attached to the camera. Treated with a common fluorescent dye, the nuclei in the samples glow brightly when lighted with the tip of the cable. In healthy tissue, the nuclei are small and widely spaced. In cancerous tissue, the nuclei are abnormally large and close together. This distortion is easy to see on the camera's LCD display. Additionally, the tip of the imaging cable is so small that it can be applied to the inside of a patient's cheek, for example to detect oral cancer. The procedure is much less painful than a biopsy and delivers much faster results.[36]

ON THE HORIZON

Mighty Miniaturization. Entirely new diagnostic tests based on miniaturized, wireless and highly sophisticated technologies are becoming part of the physician's diagnostic toolkit, with many more on the horizon. The following are just a small sample of what is under development and starting to be introduced to the practice of healthcare.

Glaucoma leads to blindness, which can be halted if detected early on. The current technology is a device called a tonometer that puffs the eye with air to determine intraocular pressure, done during an annual eye exam. Unfortunately, pressure varies widely during the day, so there is only a small chance that the symptom presents itself exactly at the time of the annual exam.

Scientists at Sensimed have created a smart contact lens with an embedded microchip that is worn by the patient and monitors intraocular pressure over a 24-hour period. If a patient wears the contact lens (shown in Figure 13) for a day, glaucoma can be detected sooner and more reliably, and the efficacy of the treatment can be monitored over time, potentially averting blindness.[37]

RFID technology has helped researchers at the University of Texas Southwestern Medical Center and UT Arlington to develop a test for acid reflux and potentially Barrett's disease. Combining RFID with impedance monitoring, an emerging science that tracks reflux using electrical impulses, the new system involves "pinning" an RFID chip, about the size of a dime, to the esophagus.[38] The chip tests for electrical impulses that signal the presence of acidic or non-acidic liquids moving through the esophagus and transmits data to a wireless sensor worn around the patient's neck. Although the patent-pending system is still in development and in testing on animals, researchers believe it will be a welcome replacement to the flexible catheter tube that must be snaked through the nose and into the esophagus, which is the current procedure.[39]

New Tests for Alzheimer's. Alzheimer's disease, notoriously difficult to diagnose, may one day be able to be detected sooner. Ultimately, doctors could predict who is likely to suffer from dementia before the progressive disease strikes, and more effective treatments could be developed and administered sooner.

Currently Alzheimer's can only be definitively detected through a brain autopsy, whereby evidence of beta-amyloid plaque deposits – considered by many to be a hallmark of the disease – can be found. There are no diagnostic tests for Alzheimer's, a disease that affects over five million Americans[40] and 35 million people worldwide and is expected to grow to over 115 million by 2050.[41] Alzheimer's is assessed by analyzing a patient's memory and cognitive functioning; these measures are behavioral, not biological.

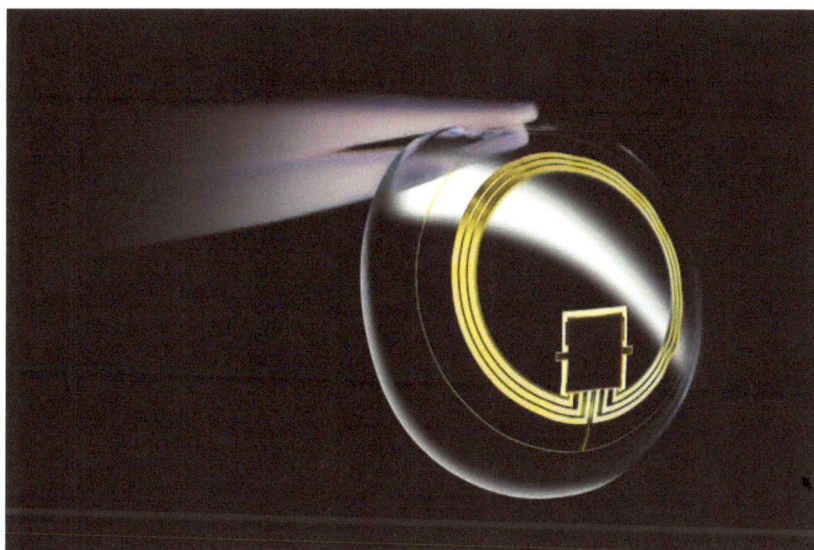

Figure 13 By wearing this smart contact lens called SENSIMED Triggerfish for 24 hours, people can continually monitor eye pressure to detect signs of glaucoma. Data are transmitted wirelessly from the lens to a receiver worn around the patient's neck. Detecting glaucoma in the early stages is key to averting blindness.
Source: Sensimed AG

Some say up to one-fifth of Alzheimer's patients are misdiagnosed, which can lead to inappropriate treatment.[42]

Fortunately, several new tests are in development that can identify the onset and progress of the disease. One such test involves new imaging techniques that detect the plaque deposits using PET scans and special chemical agents or compounds (currently in clinical trials) that "light up" the offending plaque.[43] Researchers have also reported that a spinal fluid test can be 100 percent accurate in identifying patients with significant memory loss who are on their way to developing Alzheimer's. In

Several new tests are in development that can identify the onset and progress of Alzheimer's disease.

a study that included more than 300 patients, the spinal fluid was analyzed for the beta-amyloid protein and for tau, a protein that accumulates in dead and dying nerve cells in the brain. Nearly everyone already diagnosed with Alzheimer's had the characteristic spinal fluid protein levels, and everyone with the proteins developed Alzheimer's within five years.[44]

If the new tests are approved, testing could become part of a regular monitoring and maintenance procedure. Earlier detection of Alzheimer's could lead to better disease management and effective medications designed to prevent or reverse the plaque build-up in the brain.[45]

Using DNA to Detect. Every person inherits from each parent three billion base pairs of DNA, which contain regions representing some 22,000 genes. These genes ultimately create proteins, the building blocks that perform most of the functions in the body. By sequencing a person's DNA and comparing it to the National Center for Biotechnology Information reference nucleotide sequence assembly, more than four million differences can be found.[46] According to researchers, "Some of these differences, called 'DNA variants,' are benign in nature, resulting in no measurable phenotypic change.... while others negatively alter the way protein pathways function within an individual and therefore

impact their health. DNA variants, either individually or in combination, are a significant factor, and often an outright cause, of most human disease."[47]

Genetic tests can show predisposition to a variety of illnesses, including breast cancer, disorders of hemostasis, cystic fibrosis, sickle-cell disease and liver diseases. Also, the etiologies for cancers, Alzheimer's and other areas of clinical interest are considered likely to benefit from genome information and may lead, in the long term, to significant advances in their management. At this time there are more than 2,000 genetic tests for diseases[48] (see Figure 14), but in reality genetic testing is still in its earliest stages. While the genetic test registry is the first step, there is no regulatory process for test standards to ensure test safety and consistency.[49]

Most importantly, personal medicine is in its infancy because there is still much to be learned about the connections

GENETests : GROWTH OF LABORATORY DIRECTORY

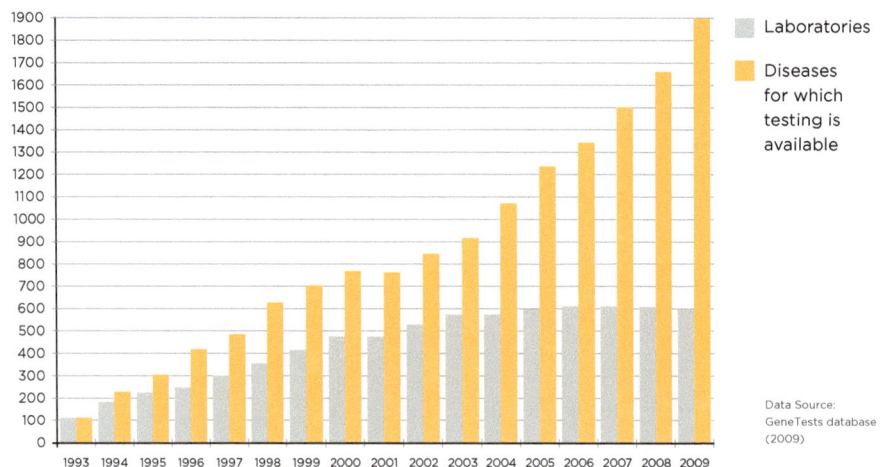

Figure 14 The number of genetic tests for diseases has been steadily rising. Today almost 600 labs test for some 2,000 diseases. (Note: These numbers reflect laboratories and tests registered with GeneTests, a voluntary listing service; actual numbers will be higher.)

Source: GeneTests: Medical Genetics Information Resource (database online). Copyright, University of Washington, Seattle. 1993-2010. Available at http://www.genetests.org. Accessed 11 June 2010.

between combinations of variants and disease. Most diseases are more complex than anticipated; it will take many years to understand the linkages and develop new treatments that will transform medicine. The last decade's work uncovered a plethora of common disease-causing mutations (variants) in the human genome, but the findings have explained only a small part of the risk of getting a disease. It now seems likely that common disease is mostly caused by large numbers of rare variants.[50]

Understanding the relationship between variants and disease requires sequencing thousands of genomes and analyzing the findings. The cost, however, of sequencing the entire genome is still prohibitive, though dropping rapidly. In 2003 the price for a complete sequence was in the hundreds of millions of dollars. By 2008 total genome sequencing costs ranged from $48,000-$60,000; in 2009 costs had dropped to $5,000-$10,000.[51]

Personal medicine is in its infancy because there is still much to be learned about the connections between combinations of DNA variants and disease.

The reason for the precipitous drop is new, revolutionary technology that is speeding the process of sequencing, improving the detailed findings, and doing it at much lower price points. Cluster processing, zero-mode wave guides, 454 parallel sequencing and single molecule sequencing are likely to significantly change the genome landscape in the next two years.

"The disruptive innovations that are characterizing this field are coming along hard and fast, and if any of these [technologies] succeed at the rate that might be projected, we may get to that $1,000 genome a lot sooner than the seven or eight years that many people have been predicting," said Francis Collins, director of the National Institutes of Health who led the Human Genome Project, speaking at the GenBank 25th Anniversary symposium in 2010. "We're going to be doing complete sequencing of hundreds of thousands of human genomes....So we have, I think, more than ever the need for a generation of computational biologists to also be human geneticists, to help us through this next very exciting phase of really getting the whole spectrum of how heredity plays a role in health and disease."[52]

GOOD FOR HEALTH, GOOD FOR THE BUSINESS OF HEALTHCARE

Breakthroughs in early detection are fundamental to the focus on wellness and health. If diseases are caught early on, they can be treated if not prevented, bringing technology to bear at all points along the way. Returning to Clayton Christensen's tenets for disruption, technologies that are relatively less expensive, simpler (easier to use, more convenient) and widely accessible will win. This is a pattern seen in the transformation of many industries (e.g., PCs unseating mainframes and minicomputers) that will transform healthcare too.

Christensen predicts that diagnostic technologies will be one of the next big business opportunities in healthcare: "...[D]iagnosis will become one of the most profitable parts of the value chain for pharmaceutical companies."[53] He stresses, "An accurate diagnosis ensures that you don't waste money and lives solving the wrong problem."[54]

A systemic retooling around diagnostics, which brings with it earlier detection, not only promotes wellness and health but makes good business sense.

HIGH-TECH HEALING

New technologies can significantly boost outcomes and quality of life.

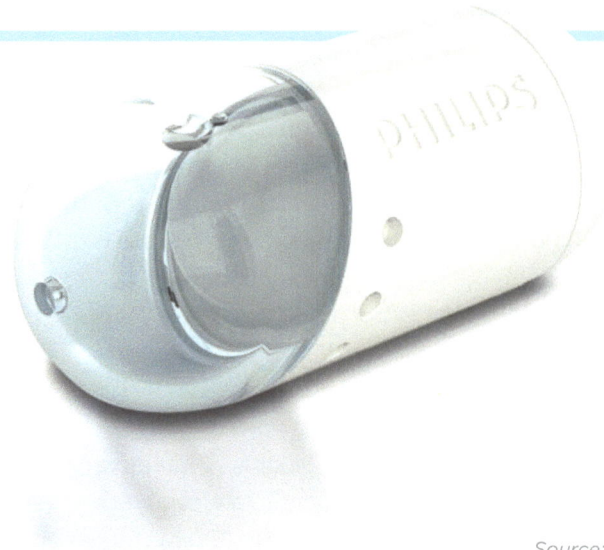

Advances in the science of medicine using technology are leading to new treatments that improve health outcomes and quality of life with remarkable and even near-bionic capabilities. While this report cannot cover all the breakthrough technologies that help the healing process, the selected few exemplify the potential to return patients to a "normal" life. The impossible becomes possible and even extraordinary as care providers have the ability to help patients correct and heal using technology-supported implants and ingestibles, the power of the patient's brain, artificial organs and bionics, and genomics.

"What we are seeing now is a fusing of technology directly with the body," observes Paul Gustafson, director of CSC's Leading Edge Forum.

"What we are seeing now is a fusing of technology directly with the body."

—Paul Gustafson, CSC

IMPLANTS AND INGESTIBLES

Technology on the inside is helping patients stay healthy on the outside. Depending on the disease or illness, the physician-prescribed treatment plan has a number of patient tasks including monitoring vital signs, managing exercise and diet, and taking medications. The less the patient has to remember to stay on the plan, the less chance there is for errors of omission that can lead to more serious health issues. The following implants and ingestibles help by continually monitoring health (disease) metrics and medication adherence – two of the most important steps for healing and managing chronic conditions.

One particular disease – diabetes – has had a lot of activity surrounding its treatment, and for good reason. According to the 2009 *Diabetes Atlas*, diabetes affects an estimated 285 million people worldwide and is projected to affect 438 million by 2030.[55] In addition, diabetic management is not a task; it is a totally different lifestyle. Patients need to closely monitor their blood sugar and make medication (insulin) and diet adjustments daily. Today's process of pricking a finger and using a glucose meter to determine blood levels is painful and not always accurate. There are problems with forgetting to monitor or knowing what adjustments to make. (Technologies that help to remind and advise were discussed in E-Power to the Patient.) The following implants improve monitoring accuracy and ease of reading (not just for sugar levels) as well as automate release of medication, both of which will increase treatment compliance and improve health.

Monitor and Alert. PositiveID's glucose-sensing RFID microchip, about the size of a long grain of rice, is designed to monitor the glucose levels of diabetics. The chip is typically implanted in the arm, and the patient uses a wireless scanning device to both obtain readings from the chip and charge the chip (i.e., batteries not required). The chip, currently in development, would eliminate the need for daily finger pricks, making it much easier for diabetics to record and respond to their blood sugar levels. An implantable glucose sensor, a vision for decades, may soon be a reality, providing comfort and convenience that result in better care.[56] The next round of clinical trials is underway.

Many articles and blogs have taken issue with the idea of embedded RFID technology because of its potential use to track a person's movement and activities.[57] Fortunately, there are other painless technology solutions for monitoring. One under development is a special tattoo that allows diabetics to more accurately and quickly monitor glucose levels. Two different research teams, one at the Massachusetts Institute of Technology and the other at Draper Laboratory, "have developed two different types of nanotech 'ink' which would be injected in the skin and change fluorescence depending on your blood sugar. Both types of tattoo would require an external device to measure and translate this fluorescence."[58] (See Figure 15.)

Each approach has its advantages. MIT is aiming for a longer-lasting detection system (six months) that would support round-the-clock monitoring. Draper's nano-bead system only lasts two weeks but is adaptable to other particles besides glucose, such as important ions in the blood. "This may make it the more versatile and applicable platform.... Blood sugar is only one of the possibilities. Toxins, oxygen levels, hormones – our bodies may one day be filled with nanotechnology regulating all of them."[59]

Another type of breakthrough embedded monitoring is the wireless heart pressure monitor, an implant the size of a paper clip that could reduce hospitalizations associated with heart disease. The EndoSure Wireless AAA Pressure Management System, by CardioMEMS, is implanted in the pulmonary artery via catheter and transmits the patient's heart mean pressure, blood pressure, heart rate and cardiac output to a receiver that sends the information to a secure Web site. Doctors can review the information via computer or hand-held device and adjust medications accordingly, forestalling a cardiac episode.[60] The device, which is awaiting FDA approval, provides more

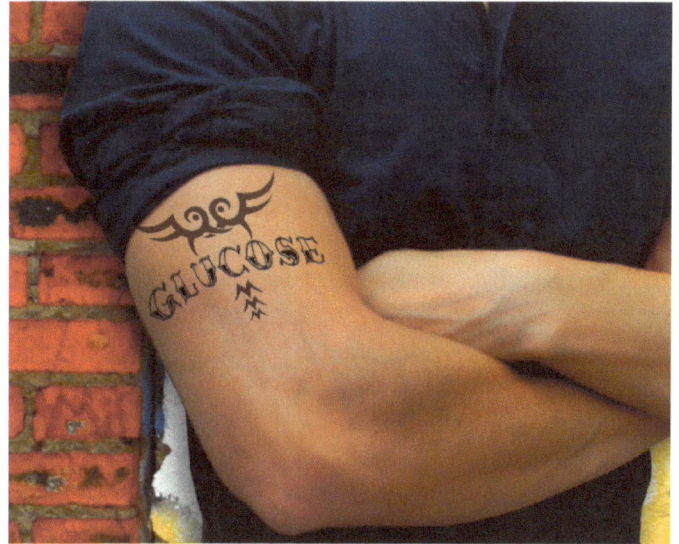

Figure 15 A high-tech tattoo uses nanotechnology "ink" to monitor glucose levels.

Source: Christine Daniloff/MIT News

continuous, richer data than in the past, when an increase in the patient's weight – a crude indicator at best – was used to signal a worsening heart condition.

Monitor and Correct. The ultimate goal is to provide a closed-loop device that monitors and corrects. That is the plan for researchers at Massachusetts General Hospital and Boston University, who have successfully completed a trial with 11 type-1 diabetic patients who used the researchers' new "artificial pancreas," which consists of insulin pumps, glucose sensors and regulatory software. This is the first artificial pancreas device that uses both insulin (to lower blood sugar) and glucagon (to raise). According to Dr. Steven Russell, one of the study leaders, "Insulin has one of the narrowest therapeutic ranges of any drug. There are also a num-

> The ultimate goal is to provide a closed-loop device that monitors and corrects.

ber of variables that affect the amount of insulin needed for a given blood glucose level. All of these calculations needed to keep the blood glucose of someone with diabetes within normal range may be too much for a human but perfect for a computer."[61]

Manage Medication Adherence. For diabetes and many other health conditions, medications are prescribed to be taken at specific days and times. Adherence to prescriptions is critical to optimal treatment and outcome. However, taking the right dose of the right prescribed medication at the right time can be a challenge, particularly for older patients taking multiple medications. In one study of adult patients with chronic conditions, only 50 percent were taking their medications as prescribed.[62]

"Reminder" solutions abound, from the talking pill box to the glowing orb to applications that use a TV, phone or PC. However, reminding the patient does not close the medication loop. There is no way of knowing if the patient took the medication. The following examples use technology to record that the medication was in fact taken, and some also release the correct medication at the right time or in the right place.

Scientists at the University of Florida are trying to take human error out of the adherence equation through "smart" pills that issue alerts when the pill is swallowed. The "tattletale pill" technology – a microchip and digestible antenna – attaches to a standard-size pill capsule. When the pill is swallowed, a message is sent to a small device carried by the patient, which in turn sends a message to a cellular phone or laptop of doctors or family members. The pill, which is seeking FDA approval and could be on the market in two years, can be used to enforce medication compliance not only in patients but in subjects in clinical trials, greatly improving research efficiency and accuracy.[63]

Proteus Biomedical is also working on an intelligent pill technology that incorporates a tiny sensor into pills for tracking medication adherence; the company, which announced a sizeable investment by Novartis in January 2010, is targeting medication adherence for organ transplants (Novartis is a global leader in organ transplant drug development and marketing), cardiovascular disease, infectious diseases, diabetes and psychiatric disorders.[64] Once the pill, shown in Figure 16, is swallowed, the sensor reports to a wearable receiver on the patient's skin (the Raisin technology discussed in E-Power to the Patient) that the medicine has been taken.

Instead of swallowing a pill, what if the dose was automatically administered? A new tooth implant in development dispenses medication in the right dose and at the right time, making adherence a non-issue. The

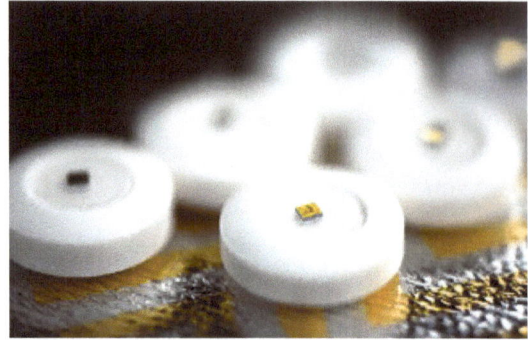

Figure 16 This sensor on a pill tracks medication adherence so patients don't have to.

Source: Proteus Biomedical

IntelliDrug intraoral drug delivery solution is a miniaturized device, about the size of two molars, that is inserted into the mouth. (See Figure 17.) Supported by the European Union, the IntelliDrug consortium is piloting the application for the treatment of addiction, with plans to expand to chronic disease management such as Alzheimer's and Parkinson's. The prosthesis dispenses micro amounts of medicine steadily, avoiding peak concentrations that can come with pills. Medicine resides in the prosthesis in solid form (a pill), mixes with water from saliva, and is released at programmed intervals. Medicine passes through the cheek wall instead of the intestines and stomach, making it easier for the body to absorb.

Because it resides in the mouth, the prosthesis is readily accessible for refilling and maintenance, yet conveniently hidden and effortless to transport. It can be programmed

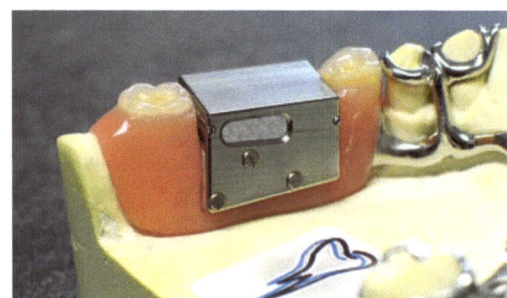

Figure 17 A tooth implant would dispense the right dose of medicine at the right time, so patients never have to remember to take their meds.

Source: Fraunhofer Institute for Biomedical Engineering

wirelessly by a physician and is available as a removable denture, mouth guard, bridge or orthodontic bracket. The device has shown positive results in lab tests with animals and is undergoing further testing.[65]

The next advancement in technology-enhanced medication management is the ability to release the drug at the right location in the body to increase efficacy. For example, Philips Research has an intelligent pill that can be programmed to deliver targeted doses of medication to patients with digestive disorders such as Crohn's disease, colitis and colon cancer. The pill, shown in Figure 18, determines its location via a pH sensor

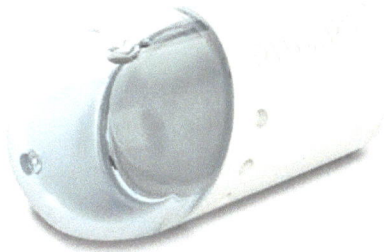

Figure 18 A smart pill can deliver targeted doses of medicine to specific locations in the body.

Source: Philips

that measures acidity of the environment. The device releases medicine from its reservoir via a microprocessor-controlled pump either in bursts or a controlled release, and can target multiple locations.[66] Further out, scientists are working on smart pills that dispense medicine when they recognize defects in nearby cells, such as DNA defects in cancer cells, enabling selective drug delivery to the damaged cells. As biomaterials and delivery systems continue to improve, having small in-body devices to deliver medications will become more commonplace.

TAPPING INTO THE POWER OF THE BRAIN

Another area where implants could have a powerful effect is the brain. The brain has long been a mystery – the subject of ongoing efforts to understand how it works. Today researchers are trying to tap into neural connections to improve quality of life.

BrainGate is a brain implant in development that harnesses people's thoughts to enable movement and communication. For example, a person could operate a wheelchair just by thinking about it or move a computer cursor just by thinking about it.

Thoughts fire electrical impulses in the brain. The BrainGate chip, a sensor about the size of a baby aspirin that is implanted on the motor cortex, captures these electrical signals as the person thinks about moving the wheelchair or cursor, and a computer translates the signals into the corresponding action. For example, people who are paralyzed from spinal cord injuries could one day steer their wheelchairs, operate a computer or feed themselves.[67] Although BrainGate, being developed by The BrainGate Company, and other brain-computer interface technology (for example at Georgia Institute of Technology) are still in the early stages, they indicate future directions for what is possible.[68]

Another type of brain implant is being used to fight seizures. The RNS System, a responsive neurostimulator from NeuroPace, detects abnormal electrical activity in the brain that signals the onset of a seizure, and delivers a specific pattern of mild electrical stimulation to block the seizure. "It's like dousing a spark before it becomes a flame," said NeuroPace's chief medical officer at a press conference.[69] The implant, about the size of a domino, offers a new option to severe epilepsy patients who do not respond to medication and cannot have surgery. The device has undergone clinical trials at a number of academic medical centers, yielding very positive results that demonstrate the implant can decrease seizures in epilepsy patients not respondent to medication. In July 2010 NeuroPace submitted its Premarket Approval (PMA) application to the FDA.[70] (See Figure 19.)

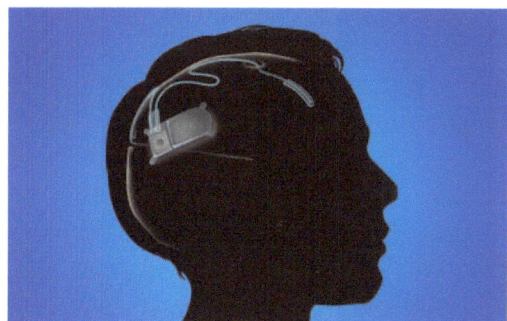

Figure 19 A brain implant can be used to detect seizures early on and mitigate them.

Source: NeuroPace

IMPLANTS SOFT AS SILK

Implants are typically made of inorganic material, so they often face the risk of rejection by the body. When they are non-functioning or no longer needed, removing or replacing them requires surgery. But now surgery can be eliminated thanks to a new implant material: silk.

Researchers at Tufts University are using silk "as the basis for implantable optical and electronic devices that will act like a combination vital-sign monitor, blood test, imaging center, and pharmacy – and will safely break down when no longer needed."[71] Silk is biodegradable, it is soft, and it carries light like optical glass. Although "it can't be made into a transistor or an electrical wire, it can serve as a mechanical support for arrays of electrically active devices, allowing them to sit right on top of biological tissues without causing irritation."[72] Silk can break down inside the body immediately or last for years, depending on how it is processed.

ARTIFICIAL ORGANS AND BIONICS

Progress in artificial organs and bionics is providing dramatically new levels of wellness. The cochlear implant or "bionic ear" was a pioneer in this field, bringing hearing to the deaf. Many more advances in development include artificial organs using 3-D printing, bionic retinas, bionic contact lenses, bionic limbs and technology-restored skin.

Researchers have developed technology for creating artificial organs on demand, using a technology similar to 3-D printing with bio-ink made from patients' cells.[73] The bio-ink is essentially dispensed into specially designed molds and grows into living tissue. Using this "bio-printing" technique, researchers at Organovo are creating simple tissues like skin, muscles and blood vessels. This is a step on the road to creating fully-functioning organs

from scratch – a vision that still faces many technological challenges.

A number of research efforts are working on eyesight, a fertile area for high-tech enhancements given humans are so visually oriented. Two enhancements are the bionic retina and the bionic contact lens.

The U.S. Department of Energy's (DOE) Artificial Retina Project, a collaboration of five DOE national laboratories, four universities and private industry, is working on developing the most advanced retinal prosthesis. To date, important progress has been made by enabling direct communication between the implant and the neural cells that carry visual information to the brain; however, considerable research remains. The challenge is to replace the lost light-gathering function of rods and cones with a video camera, and to use the camera-collected information to electronically stimulate the part of the retina not destroyed by disease. In addition, a software system called the Artificial Retinal Implant Vision Simulator (ARIVS) provides "real-time image processing to improve the vision afforded by the camera-driven device. The preservation and enhancement of contrast differences and transitions, such as edges, are particularly important compared to picture details like object texture."[74] (See Figure 20.)

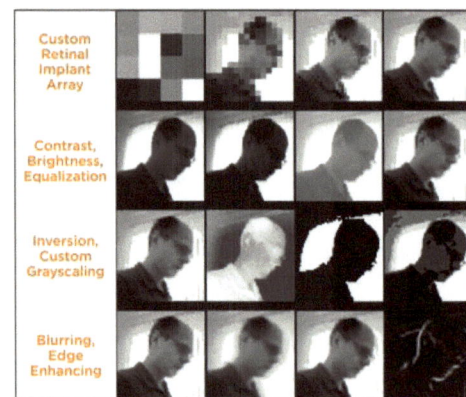

Figure 20 These images represent a typical palette of image-processing modules (filters) that are applied in real time to enhance the video camera stream driving the Artificial Retina.

Source: The images were generated by the U.S. Department of Energy-funded Artificial Retinal Implant Vision Simulator (ARIVS) devised and developed by Dr. Wolfgang Fink and Mark Tarbell at the Visual and Autonomous Exploration Systems Research Laboratory, California Institute of Technology.

Whereas the bionic retina corrects, the bionic contact lens augments. The lens packs circuitry, LEDs and antennae on an area roughly 1.2 millimeters in diameter, and has the potential for numerous applications, from healthcare to education. A bionic contact lens being developed at the University of Washington would superimpose images and data onto the real world the person sees, making it easier, for example, to read repair manuals while working on a machine. In addition, the bionic lens could monitor the wearer's biomarkers and health indicators, reporting on such measures as blood-sugar levels so that diabetics would not need to prick themselves. According to one of the lead researchers, "We already see a future in which the humble contact lens becomes a real platform, like the iPhone is today, with lots of developers contributing their ideas and inventions. As far as we're concerned, the possibilities extend as far as the eye can see, and beyond."[75]

Bionic Prosthetics. A truly disruptive technology breakthrough for people is the development of life-like, workable limbs and hands with incredible dexterity. For example, Touch Bionics creates advanced upper-limb prosthetics including hands, fingers and skin. Its i-LIMB Pulse prosthetic hand, shown in Figure 21, provides extraordinary levels of dexterity and control, using mechanical engineering for five fully-articulated fingers and high-strength plastics that are lightweight and robust. The hand has a control system based on a traditional myoelectric signal (muscle signal from the remaining limb) to open and close the hand's life-like fingers.[76] The hand can bend, touch, pick

up and point, mimicking a natural hand more closely than earlier prosthetics, and its features can be customized to a person's preference via wireless Bluetooth software.[77]

Touch Bionics also creates artificial skin that is used as a covering for the i-LIMB Pulse. The LIVINGSKIN product can be fully customized and includes nails, veins and freckles to match the living hand.[78]

DEKA Research and Development is working on an advanced prosthetic arm for the U.S. Defense Advanced Research Projects Agency (DARPA). The Luke arm enables the wearer to pick up a raisin without dropping it or pick up a grape without crushing it.[79]

The arm uses a non-neural software interface that taps the residual nerve bundle nearest the arm, though the arm can work with a neural interface should one be developed. "Think of the arm as the ultimate peripheral," said Dean Kamen, founder of DEKA and the arm's inventor,[80] at a conference. Prosthetics have come a long way, as Figure 22 illustrates.

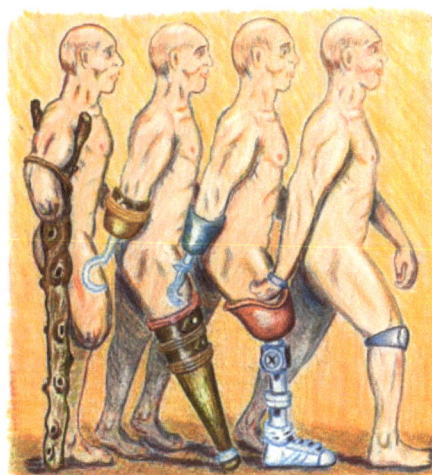

Figure 22 Prosthetics have come a long way in their functionality and ease of use.

Source: Amputee Coalition of America (www.amputee-coalition.org) By S. McNutt © 2007 by ACA

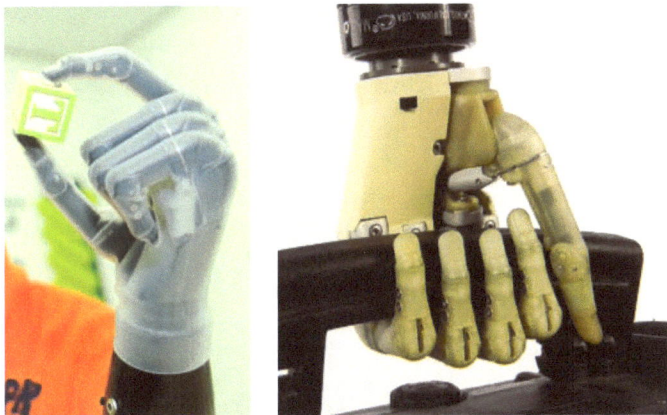

Figure 21 The i-LIMB Pulse artificial hand mimics a natural hand by having five individually powered fingers, providing enhanced dexterity and grip.

Source: Touch Bionics

The Center for Advanced Surgical and Interventional Technology (CASIT), part of the UCLA School of Medicine, is working on a high-tech vest that improves balance for patients with prosthetics or who have brain injuries.[81] Patients with a leg prosthesis have force sensors in a shoe insert of the prosthetic leg to detect foot pressure and direction. Signals from the sensors are sent to the upper leg via pneumatic actuators on a cuff worn around the thigh. The device adds sensation to an otherwise unfeeling prosthetic by prodding the thigh as the foot moves. The high-tech vest worn by the patient contains the electronics and air tank. For balance patients, CASIT researchers are working on how to signal a tilt, with a corresponding adjustment from the vest to help the patient regain balance.[82]

New Skin Using Old Technology. Scientists at Wake Forest University have discovered how to apply ink-jet printer technology to "print" proteins directly onto a burn victim's body for faster and more thorough healing. By using protein-based skin cells instead of ink, researchers can spray layers of skin that will be absorbed into a patient's body and eventually regenerate on their own. Such bioprinting is still in the lab testing stage, but results with mice show much faster healing compared to current methods.[83]

GENOMICS AND HEALING

Although the payoff from sequencing the genome back in 2003 has not produced a multitude of new healing and gene manipulation solutions, there has been progress in medication-based treatments – namely, better ways to identify if a medication will be effective, improved dosing for highly effective but highly toxic drugs, and a limited but growing number of new drugs.

Researchers have found that an abnormality on chromosome 17, called CEP17, is a "highly significant indicator" that a breast tumor will respond to chemotherapy drugs called anthracyclines.[84] "CEP17 is on the same chromosome as other genes known to be involved in breast cancer, such as HER-2, and can be detected with a simple test called fluorescent in situ hybridization, or FISH."[85] Detecting CEP17 would enable doctors to

customize treatment, prescribing anthracyclines only to those with CEP17 tumors, the findings suggest.

According to a three-year study by the Mayo Clinic and Medco on genetic testing and the dosing of the blood thinning drug warfarin (brand name Coumadin), "patients whose therapy included genetic testing were 31 percent less likely to be hospitalized for any cause and 28 percent less likely to be hospitalized for a bleeding episode or thromboembolism when compared to patients using the blood thinner without genetic testing to determine how sensitive they may be to the drug."[86] Based on this study and many others over the past two years, the FDA's warfarin label now reads: "The patient's CYP2C9 and VKORC1 genotype information, when available, can assist in selection of the starting dose." That is because mutations of these two genes affect how people metabolize warfarin, with mutations suggesting a lower initial dose.

New drugs based on genomics are starting to appear on the market. An osteoporosis drug called Prolia, by Amgen, was approved by the FDA in June 2010. In its research, Amgen made different genes in mice overactive and discovered that mice with a certain overactive gene had unusually thick bones. Another drug, Benlysta by Human Genome Sciences, was submitted to the FDA in June 2010; if approved, it could be the first new drug for lupus in decades.[87]

TECHNOLOGY AND HEALING OUTLOOK

Technology and medicine are combining in new ways to fight diseases and restore human functionality. Whether working at the molecular level to analyze genetic variants to help scientists and researchers develop new, more accurate medication therapies; working inside the body to monitor status, provide treatment, or augment or replace functions; or working with the body to provide mobility and dexterity, technology is a critical component for the future of healthcare and the patient's rapid return to wellness and a better quality of life.

RESOURCES: MORE, BUT DIFFERENT

Solving the healthcare resource puzzle requires new players and new care models.

Source: InTouch Health

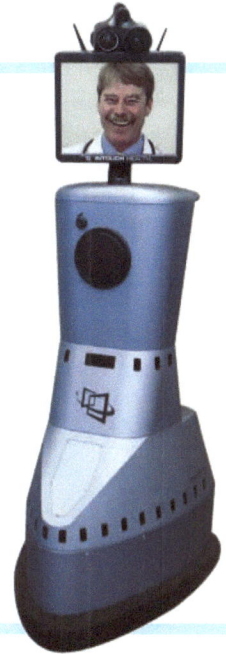

In simple economic terms, healthcare is a world of supply and demand. On the demand side for health resources, statistics have shown that there is an ever-increasing need for healthcare providers. Two major reasons for this are the growing aging population (from 2000 to 2050, the number of people on the planet ages 60 and over will triple from 600 million to 2 billion[88]) and the increasing prevalence of chronic conditions among children and adults (chronic diseases, not infectious diseases, will be the leading cause of death globally by 2030[89]).

The resource (supply) side of healthcare economics cannot grow to meet the demand. By 2025, it is estimated that the United States alone will be short 260,000 registered nurses and at least 124,000 physicians.[90] (See Figure 23.) Our medical and nursing education systems cannot possibly expand at a rate that would produce the number of new practitioners needed to fill this gap.

CHANGING THE EQUATION

The solution lies in complex changes in care delivery that offer a variety of avenues for care treatment and different levels of care providers to better match skills to patient need (i.e., to allow providers to "work to their license"). However, barriers abound for these changes. The current face-to-face physician practice model in an office setting doesn't support them. Nor does patient behavior; in most cases, people expect to see the doctor, so anything but this is a sea change, especially for older patients. Payers in some countries, including the United States, do not reimburse physicians for care outside the traditional setting, or pay significantly less.

The future of healthcare depends on radical changes, particularly those that

BASELINE SCENARIO PROJECTIONS OF FTE PHYSICIANS

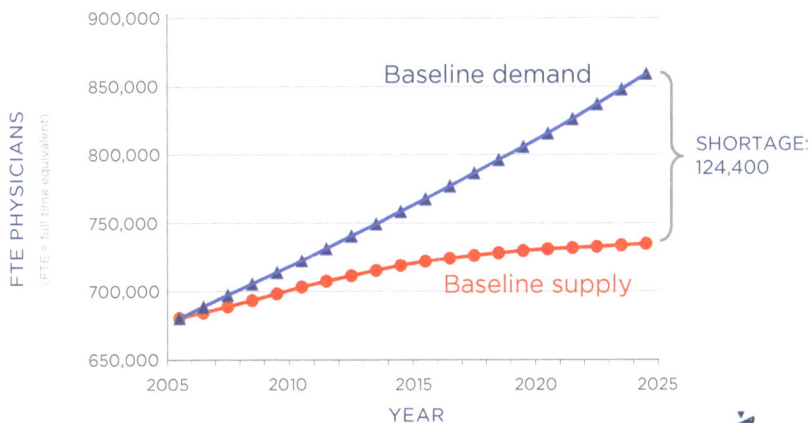

Figure 23 The shortage of physicians in the U.S. is projected to exceed 124,000 by 2025.

AAMC

optimize scarce healthcare resources while providing high quality care. Three trends are developing in labs, pilot projects and local care practices that bring to light potential approaches to fix this strained system by combining new resources, different processes and emerging technologies:

1. Redesigned care team that blends skills and technology to optimize resources and care delivery
2. Next-generation training and ongoing education to support the new care team
3. New care models inside and outside office walls

"Healthcare organizations must be learning organizations, using the data they are collecting to make changes in practices to provide better, more efficient and effective care."

—Dr. Harald Deutsch, CSC

"Healthcare organizations must be learning organizations, using the data they are collecting to make changes in practices to provide better, more efficient and effective care," says Dr. Harald Deutsch, vice president of CSC's healthcare sector for Europe, the Middle East and Africa.

REDESIGNED CARE TEAM OPTIMIZES RESOURCES

Healthcare is not a solo effort. It requires a team of individuals who provide care to patients as directed by the care coordinator. In the new care team model, the primary care physician plays a central role as coordinator, developer of the care plan, and care provider. The model is built on the principle that each team member plays an important role based on his or her level of training, allowing the physician and nurse practitioner to manage complex medical decisions. Other team members including nurses, dieticians, chronic care coaches, physician assistants and medical assistants execute the plan.

Shifting Roles. The Electronic Health Record (EHR) is probably the most disruptive technology that has helped, and will continue to help, shift duties. For example, at UNITE Health Center most of the responsibility for patient teaching has shifted to patient care assistants, who are

hired with medical assistance credentials. Using evidence-based resources and self-developed materials on chronic disease management, the practice put together a training program. When the medical assistants passed all required modules, they were promoted to health coaches and worked individually with patients. Essential to the project was the center's EHR system that allowed the health coaches to track patients and provided templates to guide their interactions.[91]

Other technology examples involve diagnostic tests that can be given by members of the care team other than the physician or nurse practitioner. The paper lab tests described in Earlier Detection can be done by a range of non-physicians and non-lab technicians with accurate results. Similarly, researchers at the University of California, Davis, have created a lab-on-a-chip for HIV testing that does not require expensive resources and is able to deliver results in seconds. Typically, diagnosing and monitoring HIV requires highly trained specialists and expensive medical machines. In contrast, the portable and less expensive lab-on-a-chip is a holographic, lens-free imaging mechanism that counts the number of cytokine molecules (inflammatory proteins) and captured T-cells (HIV-infected white blood cells) to determine if the blood is HIV positive.[92] With alterations, this lab-on-a-chip could be used to accurately measure a wide variety of blood factors for patients at the point of care at an affordable cost.[93] (See Figure 24.)

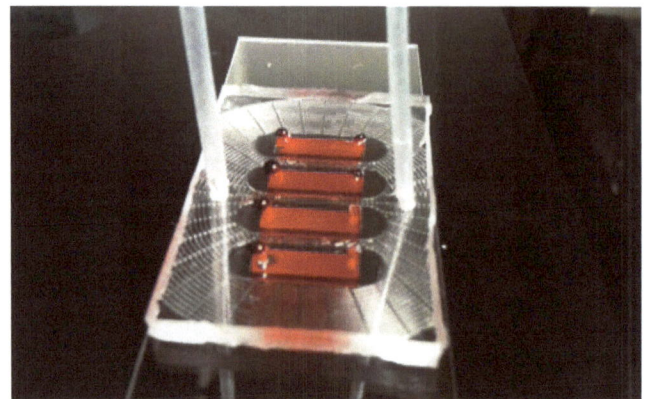

Figure 24 This lab-on-a-chip test for HIV does not require costly machines or specialists.
Source: University Of California, Davis

Patient and Family Are Active Members of the Care Team. There are more care providers in the new care team model. The patient is a member of the care team, as is the family. For this all-encompassing team approach to be successful, the team needs to stay connected so information, problems, questions and progress can be tracked and shared by all. As described in E-Power to the Patient, the technology core is a solution that has a suite of wellness and health applications. The patient and provider decide which ones are appropriate and configure them with alerts, reminders, content and social networking services to support the patient's needs. The care team (physician, nurse, coach, patient and family) uses the technology to communicate and to access and share data, as depicted in Figure 25.

Technology as a Member of the Care Team. Technology supports the care team but can also be a full-fledged member, completing care tasks without human intervention.

Smartphones top the list. As discussed in E-Power to the Patient, the biggest technology member of the care team is also one of the smallest: the smartphone. The smartphone can be a personal care assistant – always there providing immediate alerts, reminders, education and health coaching.

An emerging solution is the suite of patient apps from WellDoc, which provides real-time coaching over mobile phones, and iPads in 2011, for people with chronic diseases. (See Figure 26.) With this solution, people with diabetes, for example, can record information about their blood glucose values, carbohydrate intake and diabetes medications. The FDA-cleared software provides immediate feedback on a person's health status – i.e., positive reinforcement or advice for addressing a high or low reading. People can also access specific health information from a learning library for a better understanding of their condition. The system provides actionable information to help patients stay motivated to improve their health outcomes, which is key to changing behavior. In fact, preliminary data from a randomized controlled trial indicated that the system reduced the A1C level by nearly 2.0 points.[94] (Every 1 point A1C reduction has been shown to reduce diabetes complications by 37 percent.[95])

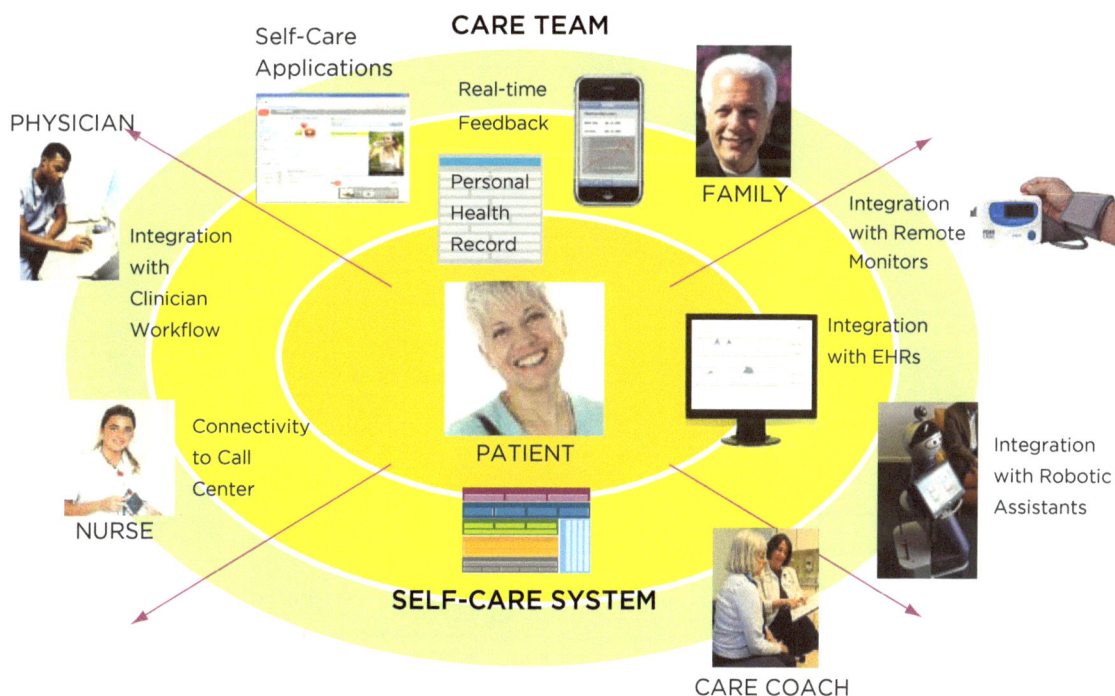

Figure 25 The care team – patient, physicians, nurses, care coaches and family members – uses technology to communicate and to access and share data. Technology itself is a member of the care team.

Source: CSC (Adapted from Chris Zook, Beyond the Core, *2004)*

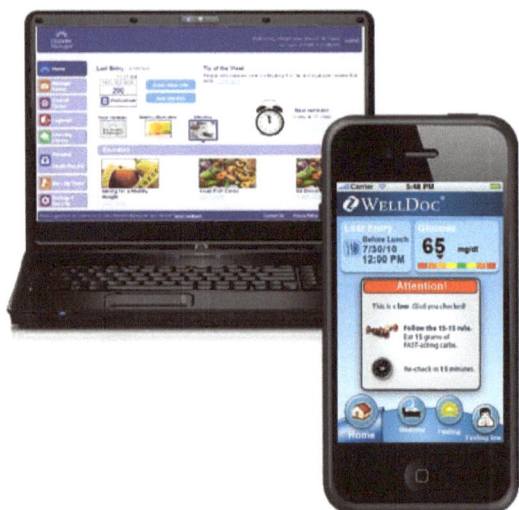

Figure 26 WellDoc's patient coaching software, on a phone or laptop, helps patients better manage their health and take control.

Source: WellDoc

Smartphones, along with the iPad and other net-centric devices, will put more healthcare information and capability at the patient's disposal, solidifying their position on the care team.

Robots are team members, too, whose role will become more prominent as the technology matures. (See Figure 27.) The Huggable teddy bear robot being developed by MIT can serve as a medical communicator. Packed with electronic sensors and sensitive skin technologies, the robot can distinguish between cuddling for comfort or agitation by sensing the strength of the squeeze. When it is fitted with audio and video, nurses and patients can receive real-time information on a child's status.[96] Another plush robot, a baby seal from Japan called Paro, offers companionship and comfort to those with dementia, autism or other problems that can lead to social isolation.[97]

For older patients, French company Robosoft offers an at-home assistance robot called Kompaï R&D to minimize the need for a home care aide. The company has released an open source version of the software development kit to encourage further development of tasks the robot can perform. Called robuBOX-Kompaï, the kit "provides functions such as speech recognition (for understanding simple orders and to give a certain level of response), localization and navigation (for going from one place to another on demand or on its own initiative), communication (it is permanently connected to the Internet and all its services) [and] automation (for personal monitoring, recognition of gestures and postures)."[98]

TECHNOLOGY AS TRAINER

With a team approach, individuals will be able to focus on specialty areas of knowledge and skills to put into practice the latest developments for healthcare. Technology-supported training is crucial, given the abundance of medical knowledge, advances in surgical techniques and the growing base of clinical guidelines. While they will never completely replace professors and teachers at medical, nursing and allied health schools, technology innovations will improve skills and accelerate learning.

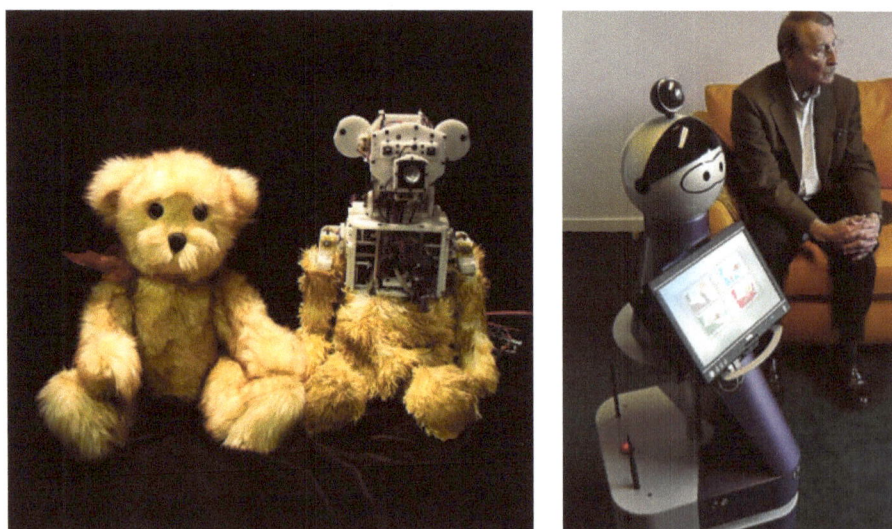

Figure 27 Robots will play a more prominent role on the care team. Huggable, left, transmits data when hugged. The Kompaï robot, right, provides at-home assistance.

Source: MIT Media Lab (Huggable) and Robosoft (Kompaï)

Medical Analysis and Decision-Making (Not Your Average Video Game). Technology-assisted simulation built into medical and surgical equipment has already shown value for mastering digital dexterity skills long before the medical student ever touches a patient. Future healthcare "technology trainers" go beyond teaching digital dexterity skills to reinforcing newly learned medical decision-making skills. Video gaming software and related devices will help professionals and students hone medical problem analysis and decision-making skills.

PULSE!! is a "serious" video game jointly developed by the University of Texas, Corpus Christi, and BreakAway Ltd., a developer of video games and simulations. PULSE!! offers professionals and students the opportunity to practice on 3D video patients using the same interactive techniques and decision-making processes they would use with real patients. (See Figure 28.) The provider sees the patient's chart, his or her physical presentation, and results from any recent tests. The patient responds to questions entered by the provider via a chat function. The provider can order tests and treatments, providing a level of interaction once available only via on-the-job training. And the 3D environment taps into the familiarity and ease-of-use of video games.

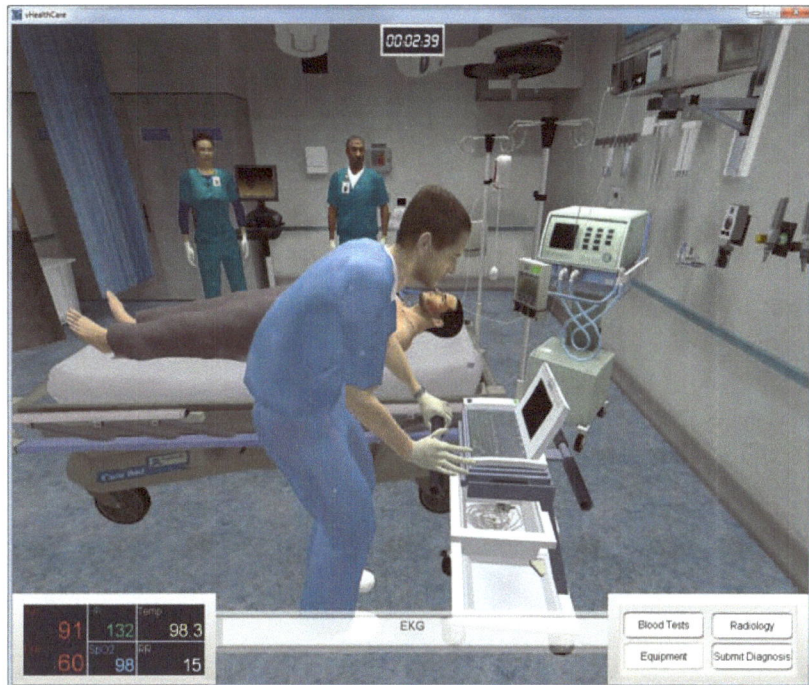

Figure 28 Professionals and students can hone their medical decision-making skills in the safety of a virtual environment.
Source: BreakAway Ltd.

Unbound Medicine's RNotes is a collection of clinically useful information for work and preparing for the NCLEX nursing exams. This smartphone application has color images, easy access by browsing and searching, and quick reference management. (See Figure 29.)

Future healthcare "technology trainers" go beyond teaching digital dexterity skills to reinforcing newly learned medical decision-making skills.

Training on the Go. The smartphone has entered the realm of medical education, allowing providers to train wherever they are. They can customize applications to target specific education needs and news alerts, and to participate in online professional communities.

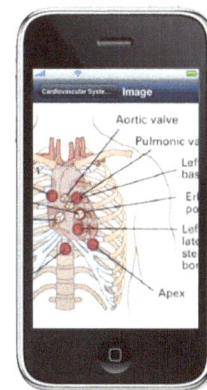

Figure 29 Nurses can study on the go using RNotes on a smartphone.
Source: Unbound Medicine

With MedPage Today, another smartphone application, providers have up-to-date information at their fingertips. The application offers breaking medical news and audio and video reports, and supports continuing education and continuing medical education (CME) testing. Providers customize the app through profile selections that include practice specialties and areas of interest. This product was co-developed with the University of Pennsylvania School of Medicine's Office of Continuing Medical Education.[99]

Similarly, the Center for Biomedical Continuing Education (CBCE) offers a CME oncology application for the iPhone. The app pulls in accredited content from the CBCE and allows medical providers to take quizzes and earn CME credits on the go. The app supports more than just audio, offering text, slides and video clips.[100] Skyscape offers a consumer version of its medical information and news feeds, in addition to its professional version, furthering the education of the patient in his or her role as a member of the care team.[101]

Procedures Consult Mobile by Elsevier allows physicians, residents and students to visualize and review more than 300 top medical procedures on their mobile devices (smartphones).[102] Clinicians can view modules in the following seven areas: anesthesia, emergency medicine, family medicine, general surgery, internal medicine, orthopedics and a collection specifically geared to the needs of medical students.

"Mobile-enabled content puts the right knowledge in your pocket, close to you at every point of care," according to Dr. Jonathan Teich, chief medical informatics officer for Elsevier Health Sciences. And it fits into a clinician's work-

> "Mobile-enabled content puts the right knowledge in your pocket, close to you at every point of care."
>
> —Dr. Jonathan Teich, Elsevier

flow. For example, residents need to track and log certain procedures as part of their training. With this technology, they can review a procedure and, within the application, log completion to the appropriate database.[103]

THINK "OUTSIDE THE OFFICE" FOR CARE

The care team approach and mobile technology allow care to be delivered anywhere the patient and provider are, optimizing healthcare resources and the patient's health experience. Wherever there is a communication link, access to patient information and the need for patient

> The care team approach and mobile technology allow care to be delivered anywhere the patient and provider are, optimizing healthcare resources and the patient's health experience.

care, clinicians can be e-powered. Conducting e-visits and supporting after-hours visits with GPS and dispatch technologies are a few of the care model changes in the developing stages.

E-Visits. Online provider-patient consultations (e-visits) can range from e-mails regarding minor ailments or medical questions, to Webcam online visits through companies such as American Well and MDLiveCare, to traveling physician robots.[104] Using online communications offers physicians a unique way to control their schedule and optimize productivity. They can work from home, work in the evening, or fill an in-office cancellation with an e-visit. This also keeps face-to-face visits open for those who really need to see a physician in person. At the University of Minnesota Medical Center, Fairview, 36 physicians are beta-testing e-visits. Physicians take shifts and commit to being available for online sessions with patients. E-visit hours are Monday to Friday 8-8 and weekends 9-5.[105]

E-visits are making their mark. Forty-two percent of U.S. physicians say they have discussed clinical symptoms online with patients, and more than nine million consumers indicate they have had e-mail communication with their doctor.[106]

For patients requiring more "personalized" e-visits, mobile robots can be the eyes, ears and voices of physicians who cannot be there in person. Robots developed by vendors such as InTouch Health and Mobile Robots allow physicians to speak directly with a patient, examine the patient's physical features such as facial movements and hand control, and determine the patient's medical problem with the same acuity as if the physician was in the same room.[107] (See Figure 30.)

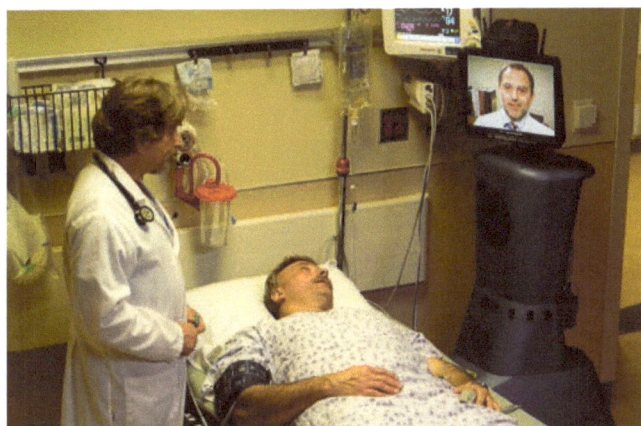

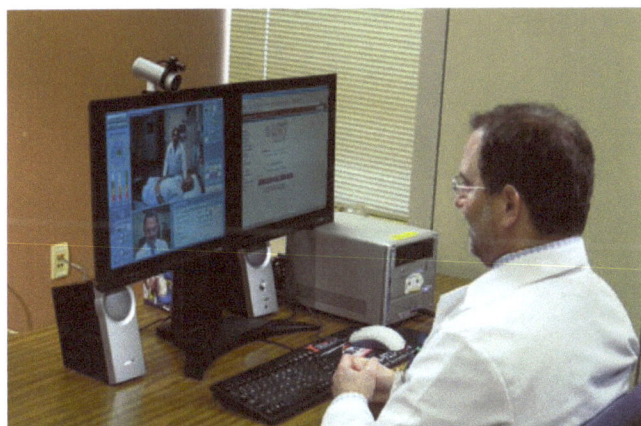

Figure 30 Mobile robots connect patients to physicians who cannot be there in person, particularly specialists such as the neurologist shown here.

Source: InTouch Health

In remote areas, e-visits save time and resources. For example, offshore oil rig crew members with medical problems can be examined using two-way video to connect to a physician. This can save a $10,000 helicopter trip to a hospital and, more importantly, provide immediate medical attention.[108] For businesses with 500 or more employees at a remote site, the telemedicine connection can be

an alternative to on-site clinics typically staffed by a nurse practitioner or physician assistant.[109]

In developing countries, e-visits may be the only option. Desmond Tutu, Nobel Peace Prize recipient and e-health ambassador for the International Society for Telemedicine and eHealth, says, "eHealth gives us the best means of providing accessible health care to the poorest and most vulnerable."[110] Care is given by care assistants and lay people with professional remote assistance, using only standard network and telemedicine technologies. For example, in Minas Gerais in Brazil, a series of initiatives starting in 2005 have created a network that supports primary healthcare and connects 100 percent of the poor and remote regions (557 villages) to the university centers of excellence, providing access to specialized care.[111]

Yet, networked villages are not common in many developing countries. Practitioners and researchers have made the most of what technology is available, with remarkable results:

- In Rwanda, volunteer community healthcare workers in the rural district of Musanze use cell phones to keep track of all pregnant women in their villages. If there are questions, complications or updates, text messages are sent to the local clinic and a response is received within minutes. Reminders are sent to the volunteers to send in monthly check-ups that are reviewed by the physician. The program has been a great success. There have been no reported deaths since the program launched last year, compared to 10 deaths in 2008.[112]

- In remote areas where there is limited connectivity, spotty electrical connections, and very sparse health resources, even a mobile phone with a camera has practical care delivery use. One missionary in Africa posted a picture of a mysterious rash on a child's arm to Facebook to see if anyone knew what the rash might be – a simple way to get more minds on the problem.

E-Enhanced After-Hours Service. Healthcare services are needed 24/7. When physicians are not available after working hours, patients often go to the emergency room. Typically the ER is not the most resource-efficient option, just the *only* option. In the U.K., there is an out-of-hours home visit service for nights and weekends general practitioner (GP) care. However, until recently the results indicated problems in many regions. The dispatch service that linked patients to providers did not have a feedback function to make sure patients received service; indeed, many missed visits occurred.

Soon, the National Health Service in the U.K. will be using the OmniLocation solution[113] developed by CSC to track after-hours on-call doctors. The solution allows the dispatcher to see both a list and the mapped location of the doctors on call, ranked by distance from the patient and required response time (six hours for a routine call, two hours for urgent, one hour for an emergency). The dispatcher is able to assign a doctor, provide a travel route and estimate arrival time. Doctors are tracked in real time by carrying BlackBerry devices to identify their location. (See Figure 31.)

In addition to accepting cases and getting directions, doctors use the device to indicate that the case has been closed – the missing link in the prior approach. In some instances, doctors also use the BlackBerry to call the patient.

As care moves beyond regular office hours and beyond the office, as the care team expands to include a variety of professionals and family members, and as technology-enabled training shores up expertise and skills, the result will be responsive, cost-effective, high-quality care. These disruptive changes are necessary to optimize scarce healthcare resources and improve health outcomes going forward. However, they will take time to absorb, and must be supported by appropriate regulatory and payment changes. ▪

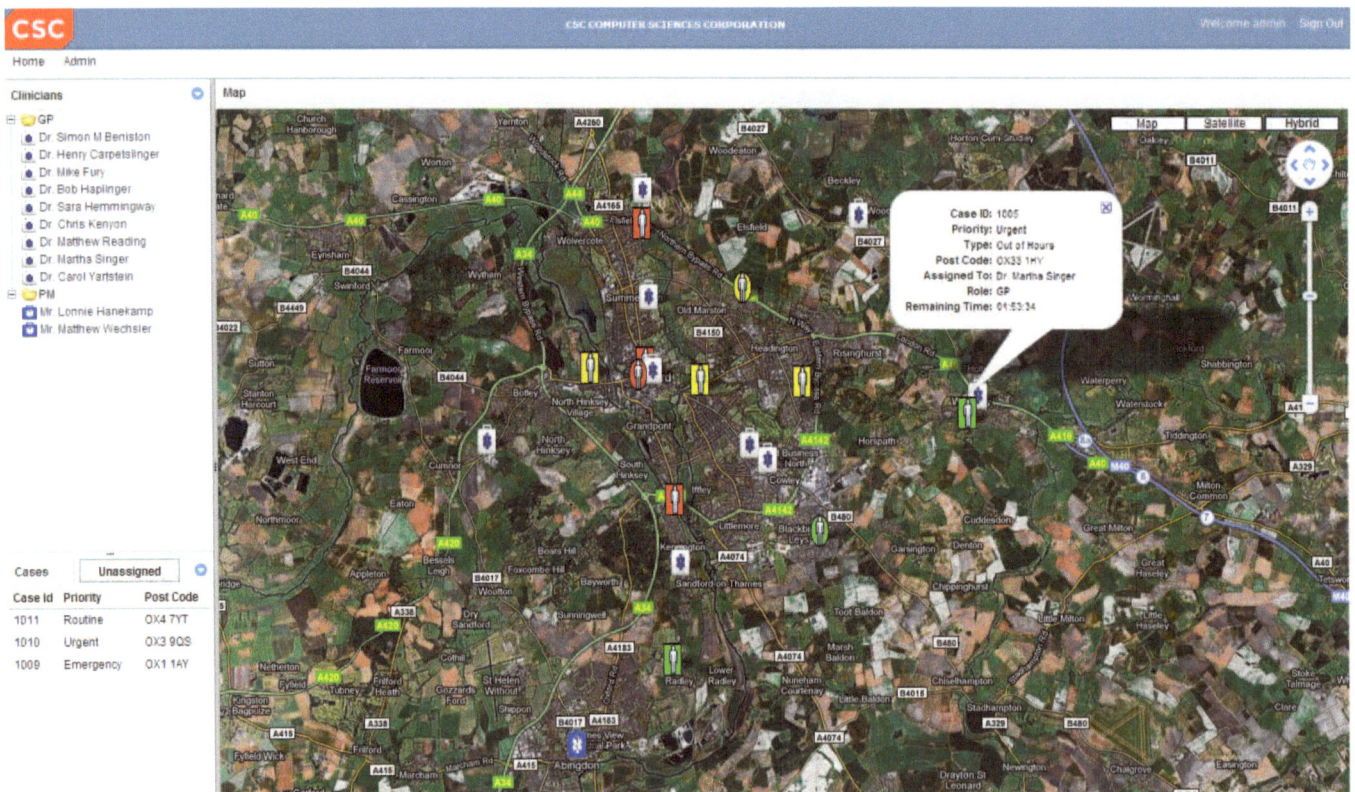

Figure 31 The OmniLocation system can be used to dispatch and monitor the location of on-call doctors. Open cases are shown in green and doctors are shown in white. As the target deadline for the doctor to arrive at the case draws near, the system changes the case icon to yellow (60 minutes remaining) and then red (30 minutes remaining). These alerts, plus turn-by-turn travel directions, aid dispatchers in getting doctors to patients on time.

Source: CSC

GLOBAL HEALTH-CARE ECOSYSTEM EMERGES

More information, more connected, leads to better care and better research.

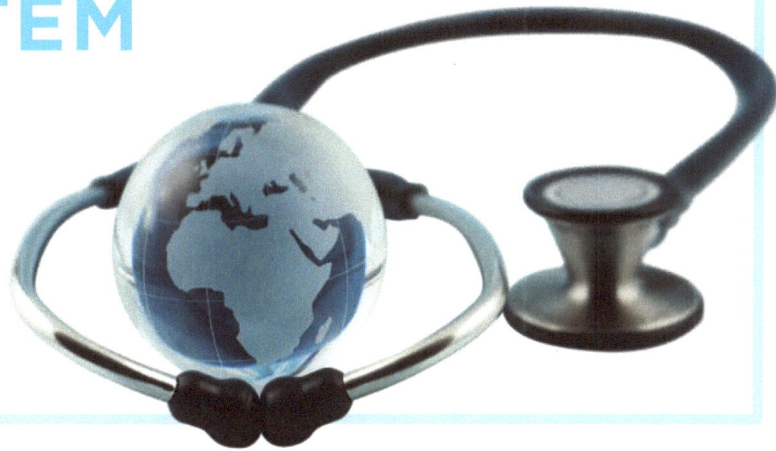

More is better. The increased baseline of information about patients, care delivery, outcomes, research study results, adverse events, disease surveillance, and population health will result in better care, and better and faster research. The emerging global healthcare ecosystem is an environment in which data are shared among the care team members, anywhere they may be located, allowing them to make the best diagnostic and treatment decisions. A network of networks, different data sources and larger populations are valuable resources to support collaborative research among care providers, life sciences companies and researchers to solve the toughest health problems. (See Figure 32.)

Establishing a global information platform is key. "My vision is a grand healthcare platform of information, where all players in the healthcare world are contributors to and extractors from this virtual pool of information," states Dr. Robert Wah, CSC's chief medical officer. "Patients, doctors, insurers, government and researchers will all make better decisions in healthcare with better information, which we will get from the grand healthcare platform. We need to turn our islands of healthcare data into a network of networks that is ultimately global."

Prior trends show we are moving in the right direction. E-Power to the Patient and Resources: More, but Different depict healthcare systems as data-rich, connected *local* environments. Members of the healthcare

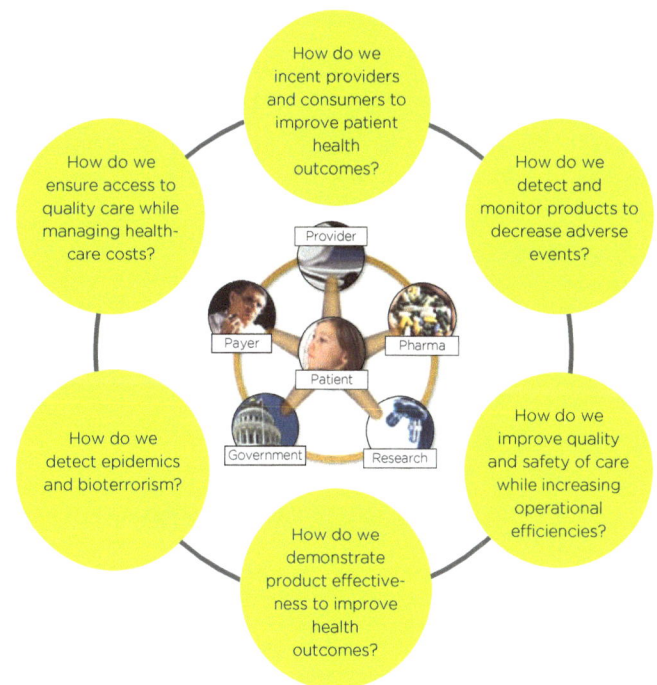

Figure 32 Increased information will enable providers, life sciences companies and researchers to solve the toughest health problems.

Source: CSC

team all contribute valuable health, wellness, demographic and behavioral data in support of patient health. In developed nations, the EHR, mobile health and wellness applications, and medical devices that collect and share data

"My vision is a grand healthcare platform of information, where all players in the healthcare world are contributors to and extractors from this virtual pool of information."

—Dr. Robert Wah, CSC

via the Internet and cellular technologies are fundamental building blocks for the ecosystem. The same infrastructure technologies and mobile devices have helped break down geographic barriers in developing nations to increase access to basic healthcare services and collect valuable data electronically.

Earlier Detection and High-Tech Healing introduced a sample of advanced technologies that will continue to extend the reach and broaden the depth of the data that can be used for advancing the practice and science of medicine. Although most of those technologies are being developed in a single organization or small group of organizations using the available data and resources, they provide fodder for the ecosystem as it matures and these technologies (and their data) are incorporated into larger networks.

Building on the infrastructure from the prior trends, the efforts described in this chapter show an ever-expanding network of resources focused on a range of patient care delivery and research developments. Information technology plays a critical role in forming this network of networks, the foundation of the emerging global healthcare ecosystem.

BETTER CONNECTED CARE

Patient Care. The purpose of patient data sharing for individual patient care delivery is clear: to expedite high-quality and safe care delivery by allowing providers to have access to key patient data to make diagnosis and treatment decisions for specialty, emergency room and after-hours care needs. A number of European countries including Denmark, Sweden, Norway, Finland and the U.K. have had success implementing large-scale health information exchanges that have already demonstrated positive results in terms of better patient care.[114] For example, Finland, which has essentially 100 percent

EHR adoption, has implemented a federated regional information system (eHealth) that supports record and image sharing and offers electronic referrals. Besides transferring data, eHealth provides a virtual working space for integrated delivery of e-services between healthcare providers. Citizens benefit from the network too. They can visit the closest emergency department or laboratory because all are connected.[115]

European countries continue to push the boundaries for patient care. The European Institute for Information and Media commissioned and published a study that indicated the positive value of data sharing across countries for the stakeholders.[116] On the technology side, the European Institute for Health Records (EuroRec) is working on consolidating the different approaches of EHR certification into a comprehensive, common set of criteria across nations, available in all the languages of the union. The main objective is to harmonize products across the union, an important step towards data interoperability.[117] EuroRec's EHR-Q project focuses on quality and certification of the EHR systems across countries. (See Figure 33.)

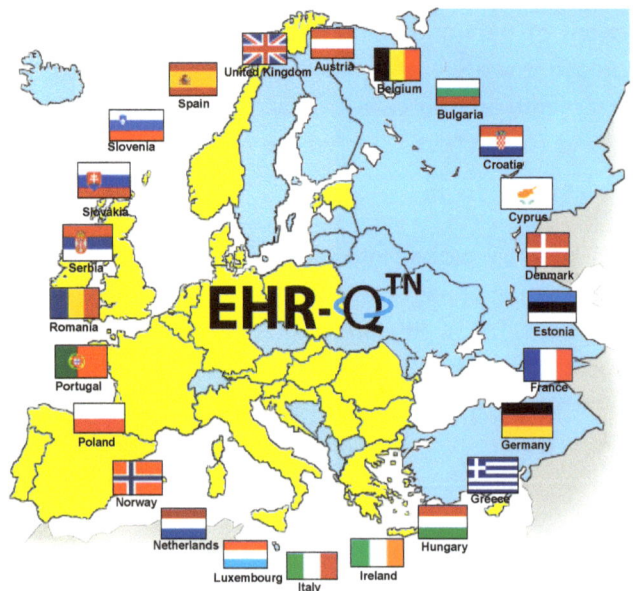

Figure 33 The European Institute for Health Records (EuroRec) is working on common criteria for electronic health records across Europe. Its EHR-Q project focuses on quality and certification of EHR systems.

Source: EuroRec

The United States is just beginning the journey to implement the foundation systems for connected care. The Health Information Technology for Economic and Clinical Health (HITECH) Act's incentive to implement certified EHR systems in hospitals and physician offices that meet "Meaningful Use" requirements for data collection, clinical decision support and data sharing is a significant step towards creating large amounts of electronic health data.[118] Health information exchanges (HIEs) connecting communities, regions, states and eventually the nation are also part of the HITECH incentives for upcoming years to support care delivery across settings.

Some U.S. organizations have already successfully moved forward on implementing both EHRs and HIEs. The Indiana Network for Patient Care (INPC), started in the 1990s to share data between two emergency departments in Indianapolis, links together the medical records of physician offices, hospitals and other healthcare facilities statewide. There are more than 30 different hospital systems, public health entities and other entities sharing data across the state.[119] North Texas Specialty Physicians in Fort Worth, Texas, has been working with healthcare organizations across north Texas to build an HIE known as SandlotConnect. This self-sustaining HIE connects 1,400 office-based clinicians and staff in several hospitals with access to 1.4 million health records and offers physicians access to information they wouldn't normally have but need to make informed decisions at the point of care.[120] U.S. information technology investment in HIEs, EHRs and population-based analytics is expected to be $150 billion over 10 years, as shown in Figure 34.

Care Surveillance. "We're entering an exciting new era in healthcare in which we have much more medical record information online. In addition to incredible value to direct

care – one patient at a time – this will bring clinical surveillance to a whole new plateau," declares Dr. David Classen, senior partner at CSC and associate professor of medicine at the University of Utah. "The next-generation clinical surveillance will be *real time* and will allow us to know when things are going well for whole groups of patients and when they are not. We will finally be able to understand immediately gaps in patient safety and quality so we can focus our attention where it can make the biggest difference."

> "We're entering an exciting new era in healthcare in which we have much more medical record information online. In addition to incredible value to direct care – one patient at a time – this will bring clinical surveillance to a whole new plateau."
>
> —Dr. David Classen, CSC

Beyond direct patient care, de-identified patient information can be used in combination with vaccine registries, adverse event databases, and pharmaceutical research

THREE WAVES OF HEALTH INFORMATION TECHNOLOGY INVESTMENT: HEALTH INFORMATION EXCHANGES, ELECTRONIC HEALTH RECORDS AND TOOLS FOR HEALTH ANALYTICS

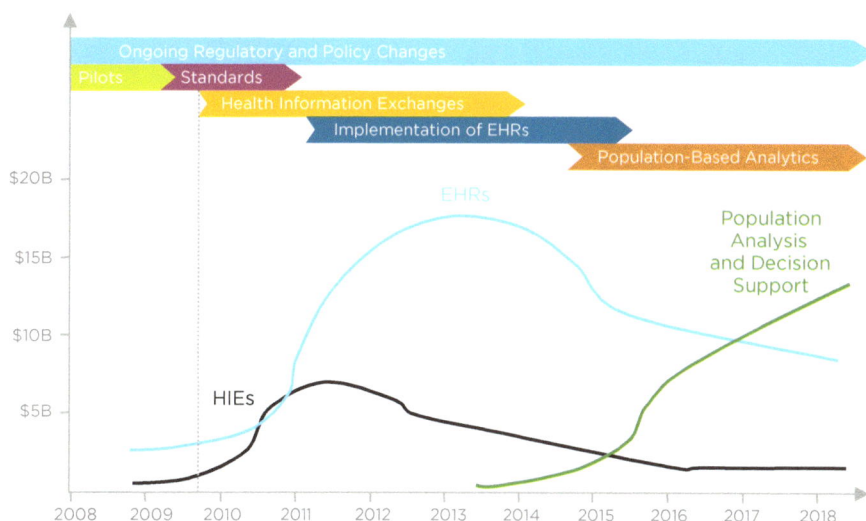

Figure 34 U.S. health IT investment is expected to be $150 billion over 10 years.

Source: CSC (2009 projections)

data to identify health outcome trends and proactively monitor the safety and evaluate the benefits of medications already on the market.

Following are four examples of surveillance organizations, their care focus and technology approaches:

- *The Post-Licensure Rapid Immunization Safety Monitoring Program (PRISM),* sponsored by the U.S. Centers for Disease Control and Prevention, built an epidemiological surveillance model to monitor for health outcomes of interest in patients who received the H1N1 vaccine. Data came from five nationwide health plans that provided claims data and vaccine data from state registries. A common data model and software for data quality check, data profiling and analysis were developed and distributed to each of the plans. Result files from each of the plans were aggregated and sent to the epidemiologists to complete their analysis.

- *The Sentinel Initiative,* launched in May 2008 by the FDA, aims to develop and implement a proactive system that will complement the agency's existing systems to track reports of adverse events linked to the use of FDA-regulated products. The Sentinel System will enable the FDA to actively query diverse automated healthcare data holders – such as EHR systems, administrative and insurance claims databases, and registries – to evaluate possible medical product safety issues quickly and securely. The Sentinel System is a distributed data network in which participating organizations will maintain control of their data but share it via standardized formats and computer programs.[121]

- *The EU-ADR* in Europe is a development project whose goal is to build an innovative computer system to detect adverse drug reactions (ADRs) by tapping into clinical data from EHRs for more than 30 million patients from several European countries. By using advanced biomedical informatics technologies to efficiently make use of the massive EHR data stored in eight federated databases and the growing body of biological and molecular knowledge, EU-ADR expects to prove that scientific and clinical evidence can quickly be translated into improvements in patient safety.

- *The Observational Medical Outcomes Partnership (OMOP)* is a U.S. public-private collaboration "to research methods that are feasible and useful to analyze existing healthcare databases to identify and evaluate the safety and benefits of drugs already on the market."[122] Stakeholders include the FDA, the Foundation for the National Institutes of Health, the Pharmaceutical Research and Manufacturers of America (PhRMA), and a number of leading healthcare delivery organizations. The collaborative, with the assistance of CSC, has built a research lab that includes a common data model, medical dictionary to enable mapping of source data to standard terminology and classification schemes, 88 million patient records from clinical and administrative sources in a centralized data base, access to additional patient records through its distributed data partners, multiple analytical tools, a shared methods library and scalable infrastructure – all accessible through the Internet.[123] OMOP promotes transparency by placing all information of interest in the public domain. A publicly accessible Web site communicates the research and knowledge to consumers, patients and providers.[124]

BETTER CONNECTED RESEARCH

There are a number of problems that significantly impact research. Work and data are siloed. Different scientists in many different universities and organizations are doing research on their patients using different methods and getting different results. Study trial populations are small and may not include the full spectrum of disease variations. Research is expensive and time consuming. It takes on average 10-15 years and an estimated $1.2 billion-$1.3 billion to create a successful new medicine.[125] As we make progress solving today's health problems, tomorrow's are increasingly tougher to decipher. Unraveling the complexities of diseases such as cancer, Alzheimer's and Parkinson's is a huge effort. For example, people with memory impairment would need to be tested for possible biomarkers and then followed for years to understand whether these markers signaled the presence of Alzheimer's.[126]

The "do-it-yourself" research strategy is being replaced by multi-organizational collaborations. A cadre of collaborations has emerged focused on a range of research areas such as accelerating the time to complete new studies, analyzing the value (effectiveness) of medical products and drugs in the real world, and monitoring how medications and other medical advances are being used to improve care. These collaborations involve multiple stakeholders that combine resources to meet shared objectives in one or more of these areas.

The greatest value of research collaborations in the long-term is the *persistence of the organization and the data* beyond a single study, allowing results and acquired knowledge to be re-used for future research. Following are four examples of collaborations in various stages of maturity:

- *The European Clinical Research Infrastructures Network (ECRIN)* supports multinational clinical research projects. ECRIN collectively represents 112 medical centers and hospitals that conduct more than 1,500 clinical studies. Presently in the preparatory phase, after 2011 ECRIN will develop as a sustainable multinational infrastructure with an appropriate legal status and governance involving the ministries of member states.

- *The Alzheimer's Disease Neuroimaging Initiative* supports data sharing to better understand the signs of Alzheimer's. Earlier Detection identified two new tests in development to definitively diagnose Alzheimer's while the patient is alive and can receive treatment – the spinal tap lab test and the PET scan contrast agent.

The greatest value of research collaborations in the long-term is the *persistence of the organization and the data* beyond a single study, allowing results and acquired knowledge to be re-used for future research.

The foundation data for these new tests came from this initiative, which was started in 2003 by a group of scientists and executives from the U.S. National Institutes of Health, the FDA, universities and nonprofit groups.

Their goal was to find the biomarkers that show the progression of Alzheimer's in the brain by agreeing to share all the data. Private companies (and patients) will ultimately benefit from the drugs and tests developed as a result of the effort.[127]

- *M2Gen* is a partnership between health delivery and the pharmaceutical industry. Started in 2006, the H. Lee Moffitt Cancer Center & Research Institute and Merck & Co. are jointly developing personalized cancer treatments for patients. Researchers use genetic profiles from tissue samples to identify genetic biomarkers for diagnosis and prognosis and to identify targets for drug development. The database combines a patient's phenotype data with genotype data. By analyzing patients' responses to specific treatments, researchers expect to more quickly match patients to clinical trials and to develop medications and personalized treatment protocols that improve outcomes with fewer side effects.[128] As of September 2010, M2Gen had more than 60,000 patients enrolled from more than 20 participating U.S. hospitals.[129]

- *The Aeras Global TB Vaccine Foundation* is partnering with industry, academia, other foundations and governments to develop new tuberculosis (TB) vaccines. The vast majority of the two million TB-related deaths annually occur in developing countries in Africa and Asia. TB is a disease of poverty, driven by poor living conditions, crowding, malnutrition and the HIV/AIDS epidemic. In fact, TB is the leading cause of death among people with HIV. The Aeras effort is focused on TB vaccines that will work for patients with the AIDS virus. There are currently four potential vaccines in clinical testing across the globe in North America, Europe and Africa.[130]

In addition to tackling the big research questions, global collaborations can address diseases affecting smaller populations because now there is a critical mass of resources and sufficient patient populations.

RARE DISEASES AREN'T SO RARE

For years, rare diseases did not receive much attention from researchers and pharmaceutical firms because the market was too small to support the development expense, and not enough was known about the affected populations to develop potential treatments. However, with the advent of health globalization, rare diseases are not so rare, and the number of resources to address these health issues has grown. Although rare disease initiatives have not reached full global coverage, efforts are maturing and attracting more resources.

EURORDIS, Europe's non-governmental alliance of patient organizations and individuals active in the field of rare diseases, has created the Network of European Rare Disease Federations. It is organized by disease (as opposed to country, as in the case of the already-existing Council of National Alliances). EURORDIS believes the new network will help to advance research and collaboration on rare diseases.[131]

In the United States, the Food and Drug Administration's Office of Orphan Products Development has created a database of FDA-approved compounds and products that show promise in rare diseases. The already-approved products in the Rare Disease Repurposing Database are unique in that they previously received orphan-drug designation, meaning they have shown potential to treat one or more of the diseases affecting 200,000 or fewer Americans. Testing an already-approved drug as a treatment for a rare disease has significant advantages. The drug has already been found safe by the FDA, and running trials on an existing drug is much cheaper than trying to develop a totally new compound.[132]

CREATING A CONNECTED HEALTHCARE WORLD

Radical changes in how organizations conduct research and provide care are at the heart of healthcare globalization, spurred on by economic realities, resource issues and regulatory changes. The willingness to share resources, to assemble new types of care and research teams, and to learn and make results available so others can build on the knowledge and experience are the foundational agreements that will lead to better connected care and better connected research.

A richer information environment is an important means to this end. This environment is taking shape as a network of networks enhanced by a variety of initiatives starting to connect the dots.

Network of Networks. As the framework in Figure 35 depicts, a richer information environment is built using a network of networks – patient information networks, collaborative research networks, knowledge platforms, and global infrastructure to enable interoperability. Together they connect to exchange and interact for specific health, disease and research initiatives. The core includes health informatics solutions with sophisticated data matching, mining and analytic capabilities.

The willingness to share resources, to assemble new types of care and research teams, and to learn and make results available so others can build on the knowledge and experience are the foundational agreements that will lead to better connected care and better connected research.

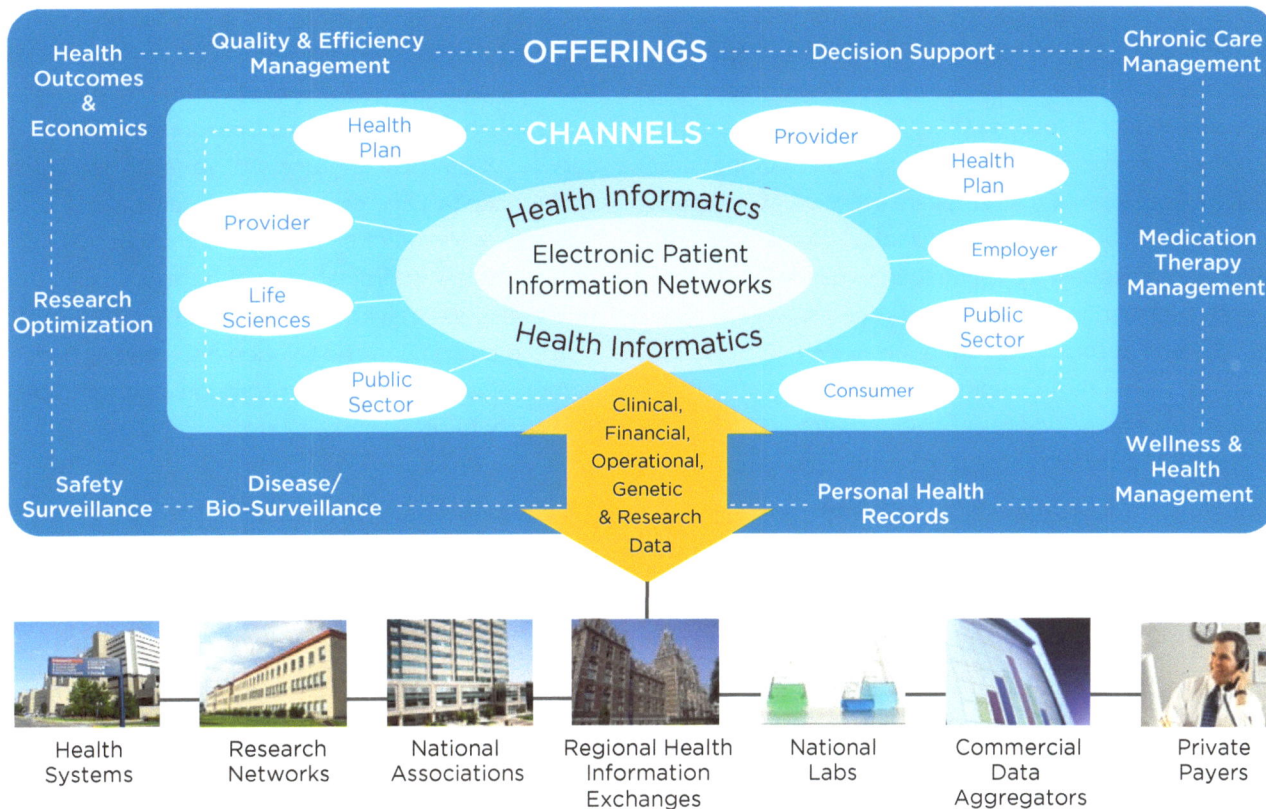

Figure 35 This network of networks shows the essential components for a connected healthcare world.

Source: CSC

The goal of health informatics is to identify trends and derive insights from the many data sources in order to make progress for health and research. For example, Blue Health Intelligence, the world's largest healthcare informatics data warehouse, provides enhanced benchmarking capabilities and predictive analytics, integrating data from 19 member companies. Designed by Blue Cross and Blue Shield and CSC, this solution contributes to greater healthcare transparency by delivering complex analyses about health trends and best practices.[133] Arkansas Blue Cross and Blue Shield, one of the member companies, received a Best Practices Award in 2010 for its use of the warehouse, for gleaning insights into a variety of healthcare trends and costs to support decision-making by employers and members.[134]

Health informatics can be applied to problems that are local, regional, national and global. The World Health Organization and the U.S. Centers for Disease Control and Prevention are collaborating on a global informatics initiative, called the Global Public Health Grid, to improve global public health by providing a standards-based informatics platform and developing a range of applications and services that leverage globally distributed expertise.[135]

Connecting the Healthcare Information Dots. In addition to health informatics, other signs of a richer information environment that is beginning to "connect the dots" of global healthcare include:

• *Knowledge Sharing Platforms* — Vendors and health providers are working on creating knowledge platforms for clinicians to use at the point of care. For example, Qualibria by GE Healthcare helps physicians and nurses draw on the vast body of clinical knowledge and best practices related to specific care protocols. Providers can both tap into information and contribute their own knowledge and rules. The platform, created in partnership with Intermountain Healthcare and the Mayo Clinic, has tens of thousands of decision support rules built on the underlying information. Qualibria is in field testing, with plans for a U.S. rollout in 2011 followed by international rollouts.[136]

- *Open Source IT Applications* — Several moves in the open source arena point towards more connected care. The IntraHealth OPEN Initiative, launched in February 2009, promotes open source software development for healthcare systems in Africa.[137] Open source facilitates innovation through shared code and broad community development. There are no software license fees, so even resource-poor areas can participate. Global-oriented healthcare efforts based on open source include OpenMRS (clinical information system), Capacity Project's iHRIS suite (human resources information system for health resources), and the OpenROSA Consortium (mobile applications that include health and research). The key is adaptability. The applications can be enhanced and combined as needed to meet country needs, both now and into the future. With the emergence of convening groups such as WHO's Health Metrics Network in the last few years, these initiatives have a forum to communicate and explore ways to join efforts.[138]

- *Cloud Computing* — The evolution of the Internet shows how global connectivity has changed the world. The next step in the Internet's evolution is to move beyond simple connectivity to deeper global capabilities via cloud computing. One area where cloud computing is aiding healthcare is data access, particularly for medical images and clinical data. For example, eMix, a cloud-based virtualized radiological image and information report service, provides secure access for physicians, hospitals and patients to view images and information.[139] In the past, this was done by setting up a special network connection to transmit the file, express-mailing a CD, or printing and mailing the image (film). Seemyradiology.com cloud services also enable image and report access from mobile devices.[140] Although in the early stages, Collaborative Care, a cloud service created by IBM and ActiveHealth Management, allows hospitals and care teams to access, share and analyze a wide range of clinical and administrative information for better coordination and decision-making at the point of care, and without investing in additional technology and equipment. The solution also enables patients to communicate with providers through a portal so patients can be more active in their care.[141]

THE SUM IS GREATER THAN ITS PARTS

Better information leads to better decisions. This is true for every industry, and healthcare is no exception. Better connected care, represented by public health efforts as well as individual care practices, and better connected research, represented by national and international studies, are the hallmarks of healthcare globalization.

Overall, health delivery will always be local, but with a global knowledge base to draw from, the local care team is better equipped to make the right decisions. There will always be a global-local dynamic at work. This dynamic will evolve within the context of the "wellness first" perspective to create a global healthcare ecosystem that promotes health, well-being and better health outcomes for all. ▪

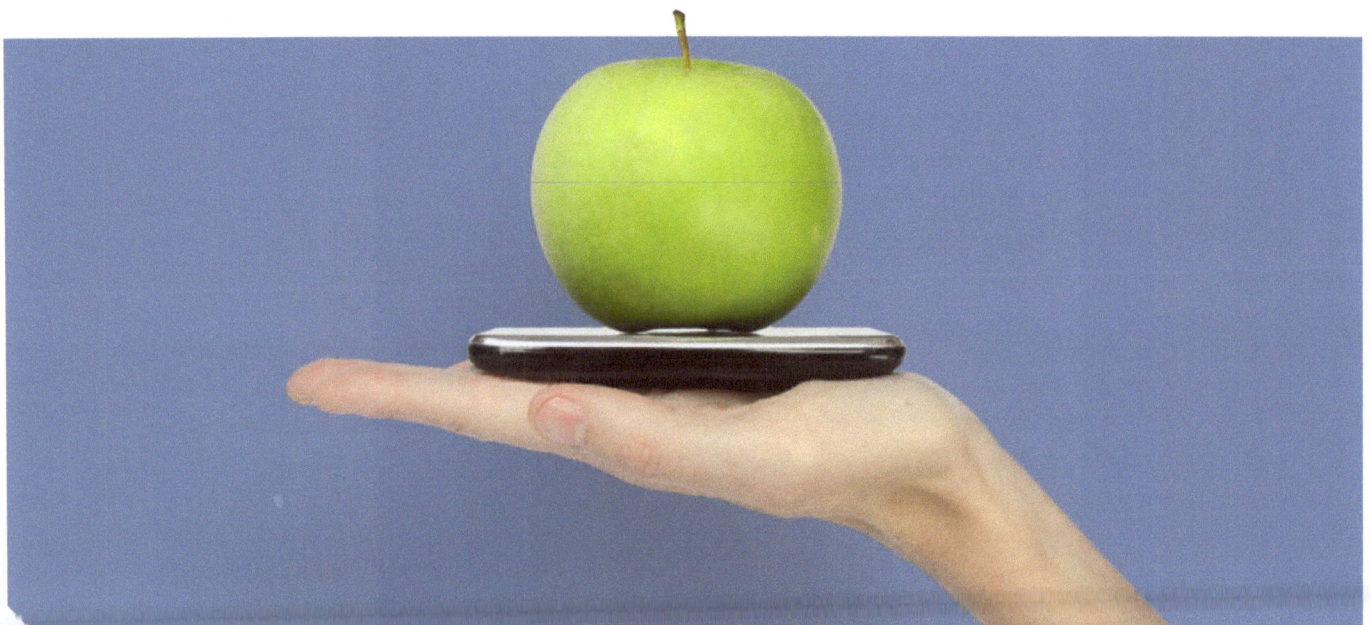

NOTES

1.   Emergence of Public Hospitals: 1860-1930, U.S. National Association of Public Hospitals and Health Systems.
      http://www.naph.org/Homepage-Sections/explore/History/1860.aspx

2.   "Testimony to Senate Aging Committee: National e-Care Plan Needed Now," Eric Dishman, 24 April 2010.
      http://blogs.intel.com/policy/2010/04/testimony_to_senate_aging_committee_national_e-care_plan_needed_now.php
      Eric Dishman is an Intel Fellow and director of health innovation and policy for Intel's Digital Health Group.
      He blogs at http://blogs.intel.com/healthcare/

3.   Life Tables for the United States Social Security Area 1900-2100, Actuarial Study No. 120, Social Security
      Administration, August 2005, p, 13. http://www.ssa.gov/OACT/NOTES/pdf_studies/study120.pdf

4.   http://en.wikipedia.org/wiki/Life_expectancy
      All the historical life expectancy statistics in this paragraph are from here.

5.   CIA World Factbook, Life Expectancy at Birth, 2010 estimates.
      https://www.cia.gov/library/publications/the-world-factbook/rankorder/2102rank.html

6.   World Health Statistics 2009, World Health Organization, p. 44.
      http://www.who.int/whosis/whostat/EN_WHS09_Full.pdf

7.   Summary Health Statistics for U.S. Adults: National Health Interview Survey 2008, U.S. Department of Health
      and Human Services, Centers for Disease Control and Prevention, National Center for Health Statistics,
      December 2009, p. 74. http://www.cdc.gov/nchs/data/series/sr_10/sr10_242.pdf

8.   Percent of Adults Who are Overweight or Obese 2009, Kaiser State Health Facts.
      http://www.statehealthfacts.org/comparemaptable.jsp?ind=89&cat=2

9.   World Health Organization, Obesity and Overweight, Fact Sheet No. 311, September 2006.
      http://www.who.int/mediacentre/factsheets/fs311/en/index.html

10.   World Health Organization, http://www.who.int/features/qa/42/en/index.html.
      Note: Most of the aging population increase will occur in developing countries.

NOTES

11.   Nursing Shortage: American Association of Colleges of Nursing (AACN) Nursing Shortage Fact Sheet,
      September 2010, bullet 4, http://www.aacn.nche.edu/media/FactSheets/NursingShortage.htm.
      See original source: Peter I. Buerhaus et al, "The Recent Surge in Nurse Employment: Causes and Implications,"
      Health Affairs, 28:4, July/August 2009, p. w663,
      http://content.healthaffairs.org/cgi/content/abstract/28/4/w657.
      Physician Shortage: "The Complexities of Physician Supply and Demand: Projections Through 2025," Center for
      Workforce Studies, Association of American Medical Colleges, November 2008, p. 5,
      http://www.tht.org/education/resources/AAMC.pdf
      Also at https://www.aamc.org/download/122818/data/dill.pdf.pdf, slide 13.

12.   Sarah Wild et al, "Global Prevalence of Diabetes," *Diabetes Care* 27:5, May 2004, p. 1047.
      http://www.who.int/diabetes/facts/en/diabcare0504.pdf

13.   World Health Statistics 2008, World Health Organization, p. 30,
      http://www.who.int/whosis/whostat/EN_WHS08_Full.pdf; and "Global Causes of Death Move from Infectious
      to Chronic Diseases," America.gov, 12 June 2008,
      http://www.america.gov/st/health-english/2008/June/20080612141457lcnirellep0.7136347.html

14.   Elizabeth A. McGlynn et al, "The Quality of Health Care Delivered to Adults in the United States,"
      The New England Journal of Medicine, 26 June 2003, p. 2635 and p. 2642, Table 3.
      http://www.nejm.org/doi/pdf/10.1056/NEJMsa022615

15.   Jean P. Drouin, Viktor Hediger and Nicolaus Henke, "Health care costs: A market-based view,"
      McKinsey Quarterly, September 2008.
      http://www.mckinseyquarterly.com/Health_care_costs_A_market-based_view_2201

16.   National Health Expenditure Projections 2009-2019, U.S. Centers for Medicare and Medicaid Services, p. 1 and Table 1.
      http://www.cms.gov/NationalHealthExpendData/downloads/proj2009.pdf

17.   "Projection of Australian health care expenditure by disease, 2003 to 2033," Health and Welfare Expenditure
      Series No. 36, Australian Institute of Health and Welfare, Canberra, December 2008, p.11.
      http://www.aihw.gov.au/publications/hwe/pahced03-33/pahced03-33.pdf

18.   "Automated at-home monitoring lowers high blood pressure, study finds," *Healthcare IT News*, 21 May 2010.
      http://www.healthcareitnews.com/news/automated-home-monitoring-lowers-high-blood-pressure-study-finds

NOTES

19.   "First Year Health Cost Savings and Reduced Risks," Industry News, The Redbrick Path, November 2009,
      https://www.redbrickhealth.com/assets/path/RedBrick-Health-Path-November2009.pdf;
      and "HopSkipConnect, now Healthrageous snags $6M," mobihealthnews, 9 June 2010,
      http://mobihealthnews.com/7874/hopskipconnect-now-healthrageous-snags-6m/

20.   "Digital Disruptions: Technology Innovations Powering 21st Century Business," CSC Leading Edge Forum,
      2008, pp. 27-35. http://assets1.csc.com/lef/downloads/LEF_2008DigitalDisruptions.pdf

21.   "E-health and Web 2.0: The doctor will tweet you now," *Computerworld*, 20 May 2010.
      http://www.computerworld.com/s/article/9176892/E_health_and_Web_2.0_The_doctor_will_tweet_you_now

22.   "How Smartphones Are Changing Health Care for Consumers and Providers,"
      California HealthCare Foundation, April 2010, p. 3.
      http://www.chcf.org/publications/2010/04/how-smartphones-are-changing-health-care-for-consumers-and-providers

23.   iNewLeaf/Digitfit Ecosystem, http://www.newleaffitness.com/QuickLinks/QL_iNewLeaf.html

24.   "New phone apps aim to boost health," *Minneapolis Star Tribune*, 12 June 2010.
      http://www.startribune.com/business/96175069.html?elr=KArksUUUoDEy3LGDiO7aiU

25.   Healthwise Consumer Health Care Decisions, http://www.healthwise.org/m_consumers.aspx; and
      "Taking Medical Jargon Out of Doctor Visits," *The Wall Street Journal*, 6 July 2010,
      http://webreprints.djreprints.com/2463100783915.html

26.   "FDA grants Proteus Biomedical 510(k) clearance," mobihealthnews, 21 April 2010,
      http://mobihealthnews.com/7343/fda-grants-proteus-biomedical-510k-clearance/
      See video of the Raisin system at: http://vimeo.com/14032810

27.   "Twin Cities hospitals aim to reduce costly patient readmissions: New Twin Cities programs designed to eliminate
      expensive readmissions," The America's Intelligence Wire, 29 October 2008.
      www.accessmylibrary.com/coms2/summary_0286-35675369_ITM

28.   Clayton M. Christensen, Jerome H. Grossman and Jason Hwang, *The Innovator's Prescription: A Disruptive
      Solution for Health Care* (New York: McGraw-Hill, 2009). This concept is mentioned throughout; for example,
      see p. xlvii: "...making it much more affordable and much more convenient for many more people to receive
      effective treatment."

NOTES

29. "More than half of Americans use Internet for health," Reuters, 3 February 2010.
     http://www.reuters.com/article/idUSTRE6120HM20100203

30. "Camera In A Pill Offers Cheaper, Easier Window On Your Insides," *ScienceDaily*, 25 January 2008.
     http://www.sciencedaily.com/releases/2008/01/080124161613.htm

31. "Just Breathe: New, Painless Diabetes Detection," *Smarter Technology*, 28 May 2010.
     http://www.smartertechnology.com/c/a/Technology-For-Change/Just-Breathe-New-Painless-Diabetes-Detection/
     This and the next paragraph are developed from this article.

32. G. Peng et al, "Detection of lung, breast, colorectal, and prostate cancers from exhaled breath using a single
     array of nanosensors," *British Journal of Cancer* 103, 10 August 2010, pp. 542-551.
     http://www.nature.com/bjc/journal/v103/n4/full/6605810a.html

33. "High-Tech Alternatives to High-Cost Care," *The New York Times*, 22 May 2010.
     http://www.nytimes.com/2010/05/23/business/23unboxed.html

34. "Paper Diagnostics," *Technology Review*, March/April 2009.
     http://www.technologyreview.com/biomedicine/22113/

35. Ibid.

36. "Off-the-shelf cancer detection," Rice University press release, 24 June 2010.
     http://www.media.rice.edu/media/NewsBot.asp?MODE=VIEW&ID=14456

37. "Smart Contact Lens Detects Eye Disease," *Smarter Technology*, 21 April 2010.
     http://www.smartertechnology.com/c/a/Technology-For-Change/Smart-Contact-Lens-Detects-Eye-Disease/;
     and "Diagnostic Contacts – A contact lens that tracks ocular pressure may help treat glaucoma,"
     IEEE Spectrum, June 2010, http://spectrum.ieee.org/biomedical/diagnostics/diagnostic-contacts/0

38. "Doctors, Engineers Develop New Wireless System To Detect Esophageal Reflux,"
     ScienceDaily, 29 May 2007.
     http://www.uta.edu/faculty/jcchiao/press_release/070530_ScienceDaily/ScienceDaily_070529.htm

39. Interview with H. F. Tibbals, University of Texas, 21 June 2010. Also see "RFID Implant Tracks Reflux with Accu-
     racy and Comfort," MDDI Magazine, R&D Digest, August 2007.
     http://www.mddionline.com/article/rfid-implant-tracks-reflux-accuracy-and-comfort

NOTES

40. Alzheimer's Facts and Figures, http://www.alz.org/alzheimers_disease_facts_figures.asp; and "2010 Alzheimer's Disease Facts and Figures," Alzheimer's Association report, p. 10, http://www.alz.org/documents_custom/report_alzfactsfigures2010.pdf

41. Statistics (as of 2010), Alzheimer's Disease International. http://www.alz.co.uk/research/statistics.html

42. "New Tools to Detect Alzheimer's," *The Wall Street Journal*, 15 April 2010. http://online.wsj.com/article/SB10001424052702304159304575184073411439884.html

43. "Contrast Agent for Alzheimer's Shows Promise in Phase III Trial," *Medgadget*, 16 April 2010. http://www.medgadget.com/archives/2010/04/contrast_agent_for_alzheimers_shows_promise_in_phase_iii_trial.html

44. "In Spinal-Fluid Test, an Early Warning on Alzheimer's," *The New York Times*, 9 August 2010. http://www.nytimes.com/2010/08/10/health/research/10spinal.html?_r=1&scp=1&sq=Spinal%20Fluid%20Test%20Alzheimer%E2%80%99s&st=cse

45. "Promise Seen for Detection of Alzheimer's," *The New York Times*, 23 June 2010. http://www.nytimes.com/2010/06/24/health/research/24scans.html?pagewanted=1&ref=health

46. Mollie Ullman-Cullere, Eugene Clark and Samuel Aronson, "Implications of Genomics for Clinical Informatics," 2008, p. 2. Originally at http://www.hpcgg.org/News/Implications_of_Genomics_for_Clinical_Informatics_2008.pdf. Now at http://www.springerlink.com/content/x33895225n282702/

47. Ibid.

48. GeneTests data as of 11 June 2010, http://www.ncbi.nlm.nih.gov/sites/GeneTests/?db=GeneTests

49. Margaret A. Hamburg, M.D., and Francis S. Collins, M.D., Ph.D., "The Path to Personalized Medicine," *The New England Journal of Medicine*, 22 July 2010 (10.1056/NEJMp1006304). Online at http://www.nejm.org/doi/full/10.1056/NEJMp1006304

50. "A Decade Later, Genetic Map Yields Few New Cures," *The New York Times*, 12 June 2010. http://www.nytimes.com/2010/06/13/health/research/13genome.html?th&emc=th

NOTES

51. "Complete Genomics Drives Down Cost of Genome Sequence to $5,000," Bloomberg, 5 February 2009.
     http://www.bloomberg.com/apps/news?pid=20601124&sid=aEUlnq6ItPpQ

52. Francis Collins speaking at the GenBank 25th Anniversary Symposium, 3 May 2010, 14:18-14:34 and 51:01-51:55.
     http://www.youtube.com/watch?v=bm7VS6FHfWE

53. Christensen, Grossman and Hwang, *The Innovator's Prescription*, p. 61.

54. Christensen, Grossman and Hwang, *The Innovator's Prescription*, p. 81.

55. 2009 *IDF Diabetes Atlas* (4th edition), International Diabetes Federation.
     http://www.diabetesatlas.org/content/foreword

56. "PositiveID Corporation Files Patent for its Implantable Glucose Sensor to Continuously Monitor Glucose
     Levels Over an Extended Period of Time," PositiveID press release, 12 May 2010,
     http://investors.positiveidcorp.com/releasedetail.cfm?ReleaseID=468996.
     Name change: http://www.positiveidcorp.com/pr/pr_111009.html
     Video: http://diabetes.treatment-info.com/verichip-now-chipping-diabetics-on-fox-news/ (2008)

57. "RFID: The Big Brother Bar Code," Spychips.com, 2004.
     http://www.spychips.com/alec-big-brother-barcode-article.html

58. "Nanotechnology 'Tattoos' To Help Diabetics Track Glucose Levels," Singularity Hub, 10 June 2010.
     http://singularityhub.com/2010/06/10/nanotechnology-tattoos-to-help-diabetics-track-glucose-levels/

59. Ibid.

60. "Wireless Heart Pressure Monitor Promises Revolution In Coronary Care,"
     IEEE Spectrum, 1 June 2010.
     http://spectrum.ieee.org/riskfactor/biomedical/devices/wireless-heart-pressure-monitor-promises-revolution-
     in-coronary. See video at: http://www.cardiomems.com/

61. Interview with Steven Russell, MD, 11 May 2010. Also see http://www.artificialpancreas.org/

NOTES

62. Barbara Kocurek, "Promoting Medication Adherence in Older Adults...and the Rest of Us," *Diabetes Spectrum*, Volume 22, Number 2, 2009, p. 81. http://spectrum.diabetesjournals.org/content/22/2/80.full.pdf+html

63. "Smart pill sends message when medication is swallowed," *American Medical News*, 10 May 2010. http://www.ama-assn.org/amednews/2010/05/10/bisb0510.htm

64. "FDA grants Proteus Biomedical 510(k) clearance," mobihealthnews, 21 April 2010, http://mobihealthnews.com/7343/fda-grants-proteus-biomedical-510k-clearance/; "Novartis invests $24M in Proteus Biomedical," mobihealthnews, 12 January 2010, http://mobihealthnews.com/6013/novartis-invests-24m-in-proteus-biomedical/; and "A Quick Look at The Status of Smart Pill Technology," Medgadget, 25 January 2010, http://www.medgadget.com/archives/2010/01/a_quick_look_at_the_status_of_smart_pill_technology.html

65. "Intelligent Intraoral Drug Delivery System 'IntelliDrug'," http://www.ibmt.fraunhofer.de/fhg/Images/SM_ms_IntelliDrug_en_tcm266-80609.pdf. Also see "Take Your Medication Via Tooth Implant," *Trend Hunter Magazine*, 6 February 2008, http://www.trendhunter.com/trends/tooth-implant-medication-intellidrug; "The Intellidrug tooth implant," Gizmag, 2 February 2007, http://www.gizmag.com/go/6778/picture/30917/; and "New prospectives in the delivery of galantamine for elderly patients using the IntelliDrug intraoral device: in vivo animal studies," PubMed, 2010, http://www.ncbi.nlm.nih.gov/pubmed/20388075 (abstract)

66. "Philips camera pill easy to swallow," CNET News, 12 November 2008. http://news.cnet.com/8301-17938_105-10095371-1.html

67. See www.braingate.com. Videos: http://www.braingate.com/videos.html Specific videos from that link: http://cnettv.cnet.com/60-minutes-braingate-movement-controlled-mind/9742-1_53-50004319.html (2008) and http://www.veoh.com/browse/videos/category/technology/watch/v17476140kmJjEhTs# (2008). Also see "Connecting Brains to the Outside World – A conversation with John P. Donoghue," *The New York Times*, 2 August 2010, http://www.nytimes.com/2010/08/03/science/03conv.html?_r=2&ref=science; and the Donoghue Lab, Department of Neuroscience, Brown University, http://donoghue.neuro.brown.edu/

68. "The future of brain-controlled devices," CNN.com, 4 January 2010. http://edition.cnn.com/2009/TECH/12/30/brain.controlled.computers/?imw=Y; and Georgia Tech BrainLab, http://www.cc.gatech.edu/brainlab/

NOTES

69. "Brain Implant Cuts Seizures," *Technology Review*, 9 December 2009.
     http://www.technologyreview.com/biomedicine/24095/?a=f

70. "NeuroPace Submits PMA Application for FDA Approval of Novel Investigational Device for Epilepsy,"
     NeuroPace press release, 8 July 2010,
     http://www.neuropace.com/about/news/20100708.html; and "Pivotal Trial Data Demonstrate NeuroPace RNS
     System Reduced Seizures in People with Epilepsy," NeuroPace press release, 7 December 2009,
     http://www.neuropace.com/about/news/091207.html

71. "Implantable Electronics: Dissolvable devices make better implants," *Technology Review*, May/June 2010.
     http://www.technologyreview.com/biomedicine/25086/?a=f

72. Ibid.

73. See video: http://money.cnn.com/video/technology/2010/05/24/tt_bio_print_organovo.cnnmoney/

74. "Artificial Retina News: Restoring Sight Through Science,"
     U.S. Department of Energy Office of Science, Summer 2009.
     http://artificialretina.energy.gov/pubs/ARN_summer_09.pdf. Also see http://artificialretina.energy.gov

75. "Augmented Reality in a Contact Lens," *IEEE Spectrum*, September 2009.
     http://spectrum.ieee.org/biomedical/bionics/augmented-reality-in-a-contact-lens/0

76. i-LIMB Pulse, http://www.touchbionics.com/pulse

77. I-LIMB Pulse brochure, 2010, p. 4.
     http://www.touchbionics.com/docLibrary/i-LIMB%20Pulse%20Brochure.pdf

78. Ibid., p. 5.

79. Colbert Report video, 6 April 2010.
     http://www.engadget.com/2010/04/06/dean-kamen-shows-off-his-prosthetic-arm-on-the-colbert-report/

80. Dean Kamen speaking at TTI/Vanguard conference, 1 October 2009, Jersey City, N.J.

81. "Vest Helps Keep Balance-Disorder Patients from Wobbling," *IEEE Spectrum*, April 2010.
     http://spectrum.ieee.org/biomedical/devices/vest-helps-keep-balancedisorder-patients-from-wobbling/0

NOTES

82.   Tactile Feedback for Prostheses and Sensory Neuropathy, CASIT research project P08.
      http://casit.ucla.edu/body.cfm?id=37

83.   "Inkjet-like device 'prints' cells right over burns," Reuters, 7 April 2010,
      http://www.reuters.com/article/idUSTRE63657520100407; "Using Ink Jet Technology to 'Print' Organs and
      Tissues," http://www.wfubmc.edu/Research/WFIRM/Bioprinting.htm (see video);
      and "New Pics: Inkjet Printer Makes Instant Skin Grafts for Burn Victims," 2 November 2010,
      http://www.fastcodesign.com/1662613/new-pics-inkjet-printer-makes-instant-skin-grafts-for-burn-victims (see video)

84.   "Gene test helps select breast cancer chemotherapy," Reuters, 25 March 2010.
      http://www.reuters.com/article/idUSTRE62O3W620100325

85.   Ibid.

86.   "Large Medco-Mayo Clinic Study Could Drive Genetic Testing for Warfarin Dosing,"
      Genomeweb, 16 March 2010.
      http://www.genomeweb.com/blog/large-medco-mayo-clinic-study-could-drive-genetic-testing-warfarin-dosing
      (Entire paragraph is based on this article.)

87.   "Awaiting the Genome Payoff," *The New York Times*, 14 June 2010.
      http://www.nytimes.com/2010/06/15/business/15genome.html?scp=1&sq=awaiting%20the%20genome%20payoff&st=cse

88.   World Health Organization, http://www.who.int/features/qa/42/en/index.html.
      Note: Most of the aging population increase will occur in developing countries.

89.   World Health Statistics 2008, World Health Organization, p. 30,
      http://www.who.int/whosis/whostat/EN_WHS08_Full.pdf; and "Global Causes of Death Move from Infectious
      to Chronic Diseases," America.gov, 12 June 2008,
      http://www.america.gov/st/health-english/2008/June/20080612141457lcnirellep0.7136347.html

90.   Nursing Shortage: American Association of Colleges of Nursing (AACN) Nursing Shortage Fact Sheet,
      September 2010, bullet 4, http://www.aacn.nche.edu/media/FactSheets/NursingShortage.htm.
      See original source: Peter I. Buerhaus et al, "The Recent Surge in Nurse Employment: Causes and Implications,"
      Health Affairs, 28:4, July/August 2009, p. w663,
      http://content.healthaffairs.org/cgi/content/abstract/28/4/w657.
      Physician Shortage: "The Complexities of Physician Supply and Demand: Projections Through 2025," Center for
      Workforce Studies, Association of American Medical Colleges, November 2008, p. 5,
      http://www.tht.org/education/resources/AAMC.pdf
      Also at https://www.aamc.org/download/122818/data/dill.pdf.pdf, slide 13.

NOTES

91. Karen Nelson et al, "Transforming the Role of Medical Assistants in Chronic Disease Management," *Health Affairs*, 29:5, May 2010. http://content.healthaffairs.org/cgi/content/extract/29/5/963

92. "New 'Lab on a Chip' Device Revolutionizes HIV Testing," DailyTech, 19 July 2010, http://www.dailytech.com/New+Lab+on+a+Chip+Device+Revolutionizes+HIV+Testing/article19073.htm. Also see journal article: Gulnaz Stybayeva et al, "Lensfree Holographic Imaging of Antibody Microarrays for High-Throughput Detection of Leukocyte Numbers and Function," *Analytical Chemistry*, 82:9, 1 April 2010, http://pubs.acs.org/doi/abs/10.1021/ac100142a?prevSearch=%2528HIV%2529%2BAND%2B%255Bauthor%253A%2Bozcan%255D&searchHistoryKey=

93. "Lab-on-a-Chip HIV Test is Quick, Accurate and Cheap," University of California, Davis, College of Engineering News, 27 July 2010. http://news.engineering.ucdavis.edu/coe/index.html?display_article=708

94. American Association of Diabetes Educators – 37th Annual Meeting, 4-7 August 2010, meeting report, pp. 59-61.

95. Holly L. Jeffreys MSN, RN, FNP-BC, "Hemoglobin A1C Value for Evaluating a Community Diabetes Education Series," *The Internet Journal of Advanced Nursing Practice*, 2008, Volume 9, Number 2. http://www.ispub.com/journal/the_internet_journal_of_advanced_nursing_practice/volume_9_number_2_8/article/hemoglobin_a1c_value_for_evaluating_a_community_diabetes_education_series.html

96. Huggable Overview, http://robotic.media.mit.edu/projects/robots/huggable/overview/overview.html

97. "A Soft Spot for Circuitry," *The New York Times*, 4 July 2010. http://www.nytimes.com/2010/07/05/science/05robot.html?_r=1&ref=science. Also see the Paro site: http://paro.jp/english/index.html

98. "robuBOX-Kompaï now available in Open Source," Robosoft press release, 3 May 2010. http://www.robosoft.com/img/tiny/CP/CP_OpSource_ICRA_EN.pdf

99. MedPage application review, 8 July 2010.

100. "Earn Continuing Medical Education (CME) Credits via iPhone," Medgadget, 16 July 2009. http://www.medgadget.com/archives/2009/07/earn_continuing_medical_education_cme_credits_via_iphone.html

NOTES

101.   Skyscape application review, 27 July 2010.

102.   "New Procedures Consult Mobile from Elsevier Enables Clinicians to View Top Medical Procedures from
       Mobile Devices," Elsevier press release, 14 July 2010.
       http://www.elsevier.com/wps/find/authored_newsitem.cws_home/companynews05_01603

103.   Interview with Jonathan Teich, 5 August 2010.

104.   "The doctor's in-box," *Los Angeles Times*, 7 June 2010.
       http://articles.latimes.com/2010/jun/07/health/la-he-doctor-emails-20100607

105.   "E-Health and Web 2.0: The doctor will tweet you now," *Computerworld*, 20 May 2010.
       http://www.computerworld.com/s/article/print/9176892/E_health_and_Web_2.0_The_doctor_will_tweet_
       you_now?taxonomyName=Enterprise+Web+2.0%2FCollaboration&taxonomyId=209

106.   "The doctor's in-box," *Los Angeles Times*, 7 June 2010.
       http://articles.latimes.com/2010/jun/07/health/la-he-doctor-emails-20100607

107.   "The Boss is Robotic, and Rolling up Behind You," *The New York Times*, 4 September 2010.
       http://www.nytimes.com/2010/09/05/science/05robots.html?_r=2&pagewanted=1&hp

108.   "The Doctor Will See You Now. Please Log On." *The New York Times*, 29 May 2010.
       http://www.nytimes.com/2010/05/30/business/30telemed.html

109.   Ibid.

110.   International Society for Telemedicine & eHealth, http://www.isft.net/cms/index.php?id=1

111.   "Developing a Low Cost and High Effectiveness Telehealth Implementation Methodology in Minas Gerais,
       Brazil," ISfTeH conference abstract and presentation, 15 April 2010.
       http://www.medetel.eu/download/2010/parallel_sessions/presentation/day2/Developing_a_Low_Cost.pdf

112.   "Cell phones save lives in Rwandan villages," CNN, 28 July 2010.
       http://www.cnn.com/2010/WORLD/africa/07/28/Rwanda.phones.pregnant.women/index.html?hpt=Sbin
       (Also see video at 1:06-4:50.)

NOTES

113. For more on OmniLocation, see
      http://www.csc.com/public_sector/offerings/11054/20217-enterprise_visibility.
      OmniLocation was developed by the CSC Logistics Center of Excellence,
      http://www.csc.com/lef/ds/22158-centers_of_excellence

114. "eHealth priorities and strategies in European countries," European Commission, Information Society and
      Media, March 2007, pp. 13 and 73.
      http://ec.europa.eu/information_society/activities/health/docs/policy/ehealth-era-full-report.pdf

115. Kari Harno, "Healthcare Information Exchange in Advancing Shared Care Regionally," *International Journal of
      Healthcare Delivery Reform Initiatives*, 2(1), 32-45, January-March 2010.
      http://www.igi-global.com/Bookstore/Article.aspx?TitleId=41719

116. "Interoperable eHealth Is Worth It – Securing Benefits from Electronic Health Records and ePrescribing," an
      EHR IMPACT study commissioned by the European Commission, Directorate General Information Society and
      Media, Unit ICT for Health, February 2010.
      http://ec.europa.eu/information_society/activities/health/docs/publications/201002ehrimpact_study-final.pdf

117. "Cross Border EHR Certification: Step towards Harmonisation and Interoperability," Dr. Jos Devlies, Medical
      Director EuroRec, WoHIT presentation 2008.

118. American Recovery and Reinvestment Act Final Rule, Medicare and Medicaid Programs, Electronic Health
      Record Incentive Program, U.S. Department of Health and Human Services, 28 July 2010,
      http://edocket.access.gpo.gov/2010/pdf/2010-17207.pdf. CSC has created a Meaningful Use online community
      for sharing information and best practices: https://community.csc.com/community/meaningful_use

119. "Indiana Data Network Provides One Stop for Inter-Hospital Connectivity," *Healthcare Informatics*, August 2010.
      http://www.healthcare-informatics.com/ME2/dirmod.asp?nm=&type=Publishing&mod=Publications%3A%3AArticle
      &mid=8F3A7027421841978F18BE895F87F791&tier=4&id=FE36164B9FC84B91A7514ED44CB5EDD5

120. "Realizing the Promise of EMRs," *Healthcare Informatics*, August 2010.
      http://www.healthcare-informatics.com/me2/dirmod.asp?sid=9B6FFC446FF7486981EA3C0C3CCE4943&nm=
      Articles%2FNews&type=Publishing&mod=Publications%3A%3AArticle&mid=8F3A7027421841978F18BE895F8
      7F791&tier=4&id=59A6223447104DAF8612A5EFFBFF3CD0

NOTES

121. FDA's Sentinel Initiative, http://www.fda.gov/Safety/FDAsSentinelInitiative/default.htm

122. Observational Medical Outcomes Partnership (OMOP), http://omop.fnih.org/node/22

123. Interview with Lyn Ferrara, OMOP project lead for CSC, 31 July 2010.

124. Observational Medical Outcomes Partnership (OMOP), http://omop.fnih.org/node/22

125. Pharmaceutical Industry Profile 2010, Pharmaceutical Research and Manufacturers of America, March 2010, p. 27.
http://www.phrma.org/sites/phrma.org/files/attachments/Profile_2010_FINAL.pdf

126. "Sharing of Data Leads to Progress on Alzheimer's," *The New York Times*, 12 August 2010.
http://www.nytimes.com/2010/08/13/health/research/13alzheimer.html?_r=1&th&emc=th

127. Ibid.

128. "Have Merck, Moffitt Found Cure?" *The Tampa Tribune*, 24 December 2006.
http://www.tampachamber.com/ci_viewnews.asp?id=1174. Also see http://www.m2gen.com/

129. "Data Sharing: Accelerating Cures," Florida Trend, 1 May 2010,
http://www.floridatrend.com/article.asp?aID=52820; and M2Gen, http://www.m2gen.com/

130. "Maryland foundation takes on TB giant," SmartPlanet, 19 July 2010.
http://www.smartplanet.com/people/blog/pure-genius/maryland-foundation-takes-on-tb-giant/4191/

131. "A New Network for European Rare Disease Federations," EURORDIS Newsletter, March 2009.
http://archive.eurordis.org/article.php3?id_article=1938

132. "FDA Database Aims to Spark Orphan-Disease Drug Development,"
The Wall Street Journal Health Blog, 18 June 2010.
http://blogs.wsj.com/health/2010/06/18/fda-database-aims-to-spark-orphan-disease-drug-development

133. "2009 Chairman's Award for Excellence: Innovation at Heart," *CSC World*, July 2009, p. 23.
http://assets1.csc.com/cscworld/downloads/CSCWORLD_JULY2009_2009ChairAward.pdf

NOTES

134. "Arkansas Blue Cross and Blue Shield Named 2010 Best Practices Award Winner By The Data Warehousing Institute," Blue Cross and Blue Shield Association press release, 23 July 2010. http://www.bcbs.com/news/plans/arkansas-blue-cross-and-blue.html

135. Global Public Health Grid – WHO-CDC Public Health Informatics Initiative: Value Proposition and Pilot Projects, http://cdc.confex.com/cdc/phin2009/webprogram/Paper21091.html

136. "Healthcare IT and The 'Connected Healthcare Ecosystem,'" HealthBlawg, 8 April 2010. http://getbetterhealth.com/interview-ge-healthcare-its-earl-jones-on-the-connected-healthcare-ecosystem/2010.04.08

137. IntraHealth OPEN, http://intrahealth.org/open. Also see IntraHealth OPEN video, http://www.youtube.com/watch?v=Pb-eJ3VJFr4

138. "Is Open Source Good for Global Health?" *Global Health Magazine*, Summer 2010. http://www.globalhealthmagazine.com/top_stories/open_source_for_global_health

139. "DR Systems Spins Off eMix to Provide Online Exchange for Medical Images," Xconomy, 6 April 2010. http://www.xconomy.com/san-diego/2010/04/06/dr-systems-spins-off-emix-to-provide-online-exchange-for-medical-images/

140. Ibid.

141. "ActiveHealth and IBM Pioneer Cloud Computing Approach to Help Doctors Deliver High Quality, Cost Effective Patient Care," ActiveHealth Management press release, 5 August 2010. http://www.activehealthmanagement.com/news/press-releases/ibm_and_activehealth.htm

ACKNOWLEDGMENTS

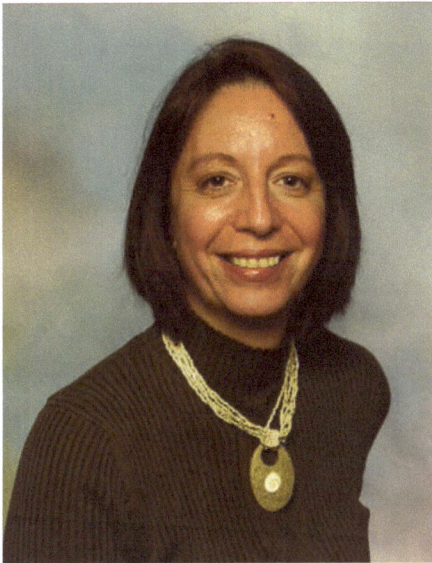

Frances J. Turisco conducted the research for this report as a 2010 LEF Associate. Fran is a research principal in Healthcare Emerging Practices at CSC, keeping her finger on the pulse of healthcare change as she leads change herself. With a 25-year career in health information technology, she has significant experience in IT systems for care delivery – clinical, financial and administrative – and research. Fran's research areas include technology requirements to support clinical research, quality measures, advanced clinical systems, health information exchange architecture and technologies, mobile computing, value and business case support for IT, and interoperability standards. She has extensive knowledge of the interrelationships among processes, applications, data and technology.

In working on *The Future of Healthcare*, one of Fran's goals was to explore the different aspects of how technology supports advances in the science and practice of medicine, especially emerging healthcare trends related to proactive patient wellness and care management.

Author or co-author of numerous papers, Fran received a CSC Papers award in 2010 as co-author of "Equipped for Efficiency: Improved Nursing Care Through Technology." She holds a BA from The Johns Hopkins University's Whiting School of Engineering and an MBA from the University of Chicago Booth School of Business. fturisco@csc.com

The LEF thanks the following for their contribution to *The Future of Healthcare*:

Steve Agritelley, *Intel*
Simon Beniston, *CSC*
Chris Bergstrom, *WellDoc*
Lisa Braun, *CSC*
David Classen, *CSC*
Harald Deutsch, *CSC*
Jos Devlies, *EuroRec*
Erica Drazen, *CSC*
Miriam Espeseth, *University of Washington School of Medicine*

Lynette Ferrara, *CSC*
Wolfgang Fink, *California Institute of Technology*
Diane Keogh, *Partners Healthcare*
Sotiris Pratsinis, *Swiss Federal Institute of Technology (ETH Zurich)*
Kim Ramko, *CSC*
Jared Rhoads, *CSC*
Mark Roman, *CSC*
Steven Russell, *Partners Healthcare*

Fanny Severin, *Sensimed*
Akiho Suzuki, *Daiwa House Industry Co.*
Jonathan Teich, *Elsevier*
Fred Tibbals, *University of Texas Southwestern Medical Center*
Thomas Velten, *Fraunhofer-Institute for Biomedical Engineering*
Lauren Vestewig, *Rice University*
Robert Wah, *CSC*